The Ultimate Dr. Sebi Enc

The complete Self-Healing Bible to Natural Healing, Herbal Remedies and Alkaline Diet. Master Dr. Sebi's treatments for Full-Body Detox and Lifelong Wellness + 60-Day Meal Plan

ANGELA HARPER

INDEX

Introduction	6
Introduction to the Work	6
Importance of Natural Health and Dr. Sebi's Practices	8
Purpose of the Book	10
Part 1: History and Philosophy of Dr. Sebi	13
Biography of Dr. Sebi	13
Life and Education	13
Major Travels and Influences	15
Discovery of the Alkaline Diet and Medicinal Herbs	17
Philosophy of Healing	20
Basic Principles of the Alkaline Diet	20
The Importance of pH Balance in the Body	21
The Concept of Mucus and Disease	23
Natural Healing and the Use of Herbs	26
Part 2: Detailed Guide to Herbs	29
Introduction to Dr. Sebi's Herbs	29
Definition and Importance of Alkaline Herbs	29
Differences Between Wildcrafted, Organic, and Commercial Herbs	31
List of Dr. Sebi's Herbs	34
Medicinal Properties and Benefits	34
Recommended Dosages	36
Methods of Use	38
Key Herbs	41
Sourcing and Storage of Herbs	44
Where to Find the Herbs	44
How to Harvest and Store Herbs	45
Preparation and Storage for Long-Term Use	45
Part 3: Diet Plans and Recipes	47
Principles of the Alkaline Diet	47
Principles of the Alkaline Diet	47
Benefits of the Alkaline Diet	49

Detailed Diet Plans   52

   Daily and Weekly Plans   52

   Sample Menus for Breakfast, Lunch, and Dinner   54

Alkaline Recipes   57

   Smoothies and Juices   57

   Main meals   67

   Snacks and Desserts   77

Part 4: Detox Programs   83

Introduction to Detoxification   83

   Importance of Intracellular Cleansing   83

   Benefits of Regular Detoxification   85

Detox Programs   88

   Fasting Guide: Water Fasting, Juice Fasting, and Fruit Fasting   88

   7, 14, and 30-Day Detox Programs   90

   Step-by-Step Instructions and Tips   92

Part 5: Dr. Sebi's Treatments for Specific Diseases   96

Treatment for Sexually Transmitted Diseases (STDs)   96

   Dr. Sebi's Approach   96

   Recommended Herbs and Foods   98

Treatment for Herpes   101

   Detailed Protocol   101

   Experiences and Testimonials   103

Treatment for HIV/AIDS   106

   Immune Support Strategies   106

   Importance of the Alkaline Diet   108

Treatment for Diabetes   111

   Blood Sugar Control   111

   Specific Herbs and Diet   113

Treatment for Lupus   116

   Nutrition and Supplements   118

Treatment for Hair Loss   121

   Nutrition for Scalp Health   121

Herbal Remedies   123

Treatment for Cancer   126

Dr. Sebi's Unconventional Approach   126

Case Studies and Results   128

Treatment for Kidney Stones   131

Diuretic Herbs and Diet   131

Prevention Strategies   133

Treatment for Other Diseases   136

Autoimmune Diseases   136

Digestive Disorders   138

Skin Problems   140

Part 6: Testimonials and Case Studies   143

Success Stories   143

Testimonials from people who followed Dr. Sebi's protocols   143

Detailed Case Studies   145

Part 7: Additional Resources   148

FAQ   148

Answers to Common Questions about Dr. Sebi's Diet and Practices   148

Debunking Common Myths   150

Useful Resources   153

List of Herb Suppliers   153

Recommended Further Reading and Studies   155

Key Terms and Definitions   157

Conclusion   160

Appendices   163

Appendix A: Nutritional Tables   163

Nutritional Values of Alkaline Foods   163

Comparison Table of Alkaline and Acidic Foods   165

Appendix B: Scientific References   169

Studies and research supporting Dr. Sebi's theories   169

QR CODE   172

Introduction

Introduction to the Work

In a world where modern medicine and technology dominate, there is an increasing curiosity and return to natural methods of healing and wellness. People are yearning for approaches that harmonize with the body's innate wisdom rather than against it. This book emerges from that growing consciousness, designed to be a comprehensive resource on the principles and practices championed by Dr. Sebi, a pioneer in natural health and holistic healing.

Dr. Sebi, whose full name was Alfredo Bowman, was an herbalist and self-proclaimed healer who captured the attention of many with his unique approach to health. He asserted that a diet rich in alkaline foods and natural herbs could prevent and even cure diseases that conventional medicine struggled to manage. His work is not just a collection of remedies but a profound philosophy that challenges the very foundation of contemporary health paradigms. The essence of his teachings revolves around the concept of an alkaline diet and the detoxification of the body to restore balance and vitality. The journey into the world of Dr. Sebi is both fascinating and transformative. His ideas were shaped by a diverse array of influences, from his native Honduras to the broader African diaspora. He wove these threads into a tapestry that speaks to the universal human quest for health, longevity, and well-being. The alkaline diet, central to his teachings, is based on the idea that certain foods can maintain the body's optimal pH level, thereby fostering an environment where disease cannot thrive. This approach is in stark contrast to the acid-forming diets prevalent in the modern world, which are often implicated in chronic illnesses and systemic inflammation.

Understanding Dr. Sebi's practices necessitates an appreciation of his broader philosophy. He viewed the body as an electrical entity, requiring foods that are naturally electric to function optimally. This perspective, though unconventional, invites us to rethink our relationship with food and health. It encourages a shift from processed, artificial foods to those that are natural and nutrient-dense. This book endeavors to make this philosophy accessible, offering insights and practical guidance for those seeking to embrace a lifestyle aligned with these principles.

The decision to compile an encyclopedia of Dr. Sebi's work stems from the need to preserve and disseminate his teachings in a comprehensive and organized manner. While his ideas have been widely discussed and shared, there remains a lack of structured resources that delve deeply into the various aspects of his approach. This book seeks to fill that gap, serving as a definitive guide for both novices and those familiar with his work. It aims to demystify his practices, making them approachable and applicable in everyday life. One of the compelling aspects of Dr. Sebi's work is its focus on empowerment. He believed that individuals could take control of their health through informed choices and natural remedies. This book is not merely a collection of recipes or a manual of herbal treatments; it is an invitation to embark on a journey of self-discovery and empowerment. By understanding the principles underlying Dr. Sebi's approach, readers can make informed decisions about their health and well-being.

Dr. Sebi's emphasis on natural health is particularly relevant in today's context, where there is a growing awareness of the limitations and side effects of conventional medicine. Antibiotics, while life-saving, are often overprescribed and can lead to resistant strains of bacteria. Prescription medications can have a range of side effects that sometimes exacerbate the very conditions they aim to treat. In contrast, Dr. Sebi's approach, which prioritizes prevention and the body's natural ability to heal, offers a refreshing and holistic alternative.

The importance of natural health cannot be overstated. It is not just about treating symptoms but about addressing the root causes of illness. This holistic perspective considers the interconnectedness of the body, mind, and spirit. It recognizes that true health encompasses physical vitality, mental clarity, and emotional balance. Dr. Sebi's practices are designed to nurture this holistic health, using nature's bounty to restore and maintain balance. The purpose of this book extends beyond merely chronicling Dr. Sebi's life and teachings. It aims to inspire a shift towards a more mindful and health-conscious way of living. It is a call to return to the wisdom of nature, to the healing power of plants, and to the simplicity of an alkaline diet. By integrating these principles into our lives, we can cultivate a state of health that is both vibrant and resilient.

In exploring the foundations of Dr. Sebi's work, this book sets the stage for a deeper dive into the specific herbs, diet plans, and treatment protocols that form the core of his approach. It provides a context for understanding why these practices are effective and how they can be incorporated into daily life. Whether you are new to the concept of natural health or looking to deepen your understanding, this book offers a wealth of knowledge and practical tools to support your journey.

Dr. Sebi's legacy is one of healing, empowerment, and a profound respect for nature. His teachings remind us that health is not a static state but a dynamic process that requires continual attention and care. By embracing the principles outlined in this book, readers can embark on a path towards greater health and vitality, grounded in the wisdom of one of the most influential natural healers of our time.

Importance of Natural Health and Dr. Sebi's Practices

In the bustling, fast-paced environment of the modern world, it is easy to overlook the importance of natural health. Every day, we are bombarded with advertisements for quick fixes, pharmaceutical solutions, and processed foods that promise convenience but often lead to long-term health issues. Amidst this noise, the voice of Dr. Sebi stands out, advocating for a return to nature, simplicity, and balance. His practices emphasize the healing power inherent in the natural world and challenge us to rethink our approach to health and wellness.

Dr. Sebi's emphasis on natural health is rooted in the belief that the body has an innate ability to heal itself when provided with the right conditions. This principle is a cornerstone of many traditional healing systems, yet it is often overlooked in favor of more invasive medical interventions. Dr. Sebi championed the idea that by consuming alkaline foods and using natural herbs, we can create an internal environment conducive to health. This approach is not just about addressing symptoms but about fostering a holistic sense of well-being.

The importance of natural health extends beyond individual wellness; it also has profound implications for society as a whole. As chronic diseases such as diabetes, heart disease, and cancer become increasingly prevalent, the burden on healthcare systems grows heavier. These conditions often stem from lifestyle choices, particularly diet, and can be mitigated through preventive measures rooted in natural health principles. Dr. Sebi's practices offer a roadmap to reducing this burden by promoting dietary habits and lifestyle changes that support long-term health.

One of the most compelling aspects of Dr. Sebi's approach is its focus on prevention. In a healthcare landscape that often prioritizes treatment over prevention, his philosophy is refreshingly proactive. By maintaining an alkaline diet, individuals can prevent the accumulation of toxins and the onset of disease. This preventive approach is particularly important in a time when many are looking for sustainable ways to manage their health and avoid the side effects associated with pharmaceutical treatments.

Moreover, Dr. Sebi's practices highlight the interconnectedness of diet and disease. He posited that many health issues stem from an imbalance in the body's pH levels, caused by the consumption of acidic foods. By advocating for an alkaline diet, he underscored the need to align our dietary habits with our body's natural chemistry. This perspective invites us to consider the long-term impact of our food choices and encourages a diet rich in fresh, natural ingredients. The benefits of natural health are multifaceted. On a physical level, adopting a diet that aligns with Dr. Sebi's principles can lead to increased energy, improved digestion, and a stronger immune system. These benefits are the result of nourishing the body with foods that are high in essential nutrients and free from harmful additives. On a mental level, the clarity and focus that come from a well-nourished body can enhance overall quality of life. Furthermore, the emotional balance that often accompanies physical health can lead to greater resilience and well-being.

Dr. Sebi's practices also emphasize the importance of detoxification. In our modern environment, exposure to toxins is almost unavoidable, whether from pollutants in the air, chemicals in our food, or stress in our daily lives. Detoxification, according to Dr. Sebi, is crucial for removing these impurities and restoring the body to its natural state. Regular detoxification can help to reset the body, improve metabolic function, and enhance the absorption of nutrients. This process is an integral part of maintaining long-term health and preventing chronic diseases.

Beyond the physical and physiological benefits, there is a profound spiritual dimension to Dr. Sebi's practices. He viewed the body as a temple, deserving of the utmost care and respect. This holistic approach encourages a deeper connection with oneself and with nature. By consuming foods that are closer to their natural state, individuals can cultivate a sense of harmony and balance that transcends physical health. This spiritual aspect of natural health is often overlooked in conventional medical discourse but is central to Dr. Sebi's philosophy. The emphasis on natural health also aligns with broader environmental and ethical considerations. A diet based on natural, plant-based foods is more sustainable and has a lower environmental impact than one that relies heavily on animal products and processed foods. This alignment with ecological principles reinforces the idea that what is good for our bodies is also good for the planet. Dr. Sebi's practices thus encourage a lifestyle that is not only healthful but also mindful of our impact on the world around us.

Another significant aspect of Dr. Sebi's work is its accessibility. Unlike many medical treatments that require expensive procedures or medications, his practices rely on readily available natural resources. This accessibility makes natural health an attainable goal for people from all walks of life, promoting equity in health and wellness. By focusing on simple, natural solutions, Dr. Sebi democratized health care, making it possible for individuals to take control of their well-being regardless of their socioeconomic status.

Dr. Sebi's practices are also a testament to the power of traditional knowledge and indigenous wisdom. In an era dominated by scientific and technological advances, there is a tendency to dismiss or undervalue traditional practices. However, Dr. Sebi's success stories and testimonials reveal the enduring relevance of these time-honored approaches. His work reminds us that modern health solutions can coexist with, and even be enriched by, the wisdom of our ancestors. In embracing natural health, we are called to adopt a more conscious and intentional way of living. This involves not only changing our diets but also rethinking our relationship with the environment, our bodies, and our communities. It is a holistic approach that recognizes the complexity and interconnectedness of all aspects of life. Dr. Sebi's practices offer a pathway to this more integrated and mindful way of being, encouraging us to live in a manner that is both healthful and harmonious.

Ultimately, the importance of natural health and Dr. Sebi's practices lies in their potential to transform lives. By returning to nature and embracing its gifts, we can reclaim our health, vitality, and sense of purpose. This book is an invitation to explore these practices, to understand their profound impact, and to integrate them into our lives. It is a call to action for those seeking a healthier, more balanced, and more fulfilling way of living. Through the principles and practices outlined in this work, we can embark on a journey towards greater well-being and a deeper connection with the natural world.

Purpose of the Book

The purpose of this book is multifaceted, aiming to serve as a comprehensive guide and a source of inspiration for those seeking a healthier, more balanced way of life through the principles and practices advocated by Dr. Sebi. At its core, the book seeks to illuminate the path to wellness by harnessing the power of natural remedies and dietary choices that align with the body's intrinsic healing capabilities. This endeavor is not merely an academic exercise but a call to action, encouraging readers to embark on a transformative journey toward optimal health and well-being.

Dr. Sebi's teachings have garnered significant attention due to their unique approach to health and their departure from conventional medical practices. This book aims to distill his wisdom into an accessible format that empowers individuals to take control of their health. By providing detailed explanations, practical advice, and real-life examples, the book aspires to bridge the gap between curiosity and actionable knowledge, making the principles of natural health both understandable and achievable.

One of the primary goals of this book is to educate readers about the importance of maintaining an alkaline diet. Dr. Sebi's philosophy hinges on the idea that an acidic internal environment is conducive to disease, whereas an alkaline state fosters health and vitality. This book will delve into the science behind this concept, elucidating how the foods we consume can impact our body's pH balance and, by extension, our overall health. By equipping readers with this knowledge, the book aims to inspire a shift in dietary habits that can lead to profound health benefits.

Another crucial purpose of the book is to demystify the use of herbs in promoting health. Dr. Sebi was a fervent advocate for the healing power of natural herbs, which he believed could address a wide range of health issues without the side effects often associated with pharmaceutical drugs. This book will provide an in-depth exploration of various herbs that Dr. Sebi championed, detailing their properties, uses, and benefits. Through this, readers will gain the confidence and understanding needed to incorporate these natural remedies into their own health routines.

Empowerment is a central theme of this book. In an era where healthcare can often seem inaccessible or overwhelming, Dr. Sebi's teachings offer a refreshing perspective that emphasizes self-reliance and personal agency. The book aims to empower readers by showing them that they have the tools and knowledge necessary to improve their health. This sense of empowerment is not just about individual well-being; it also extends to a broader societal impact, as more people embracing natural health practices can lead to a collective improvement in public health.

Furthermore, this book seeks to honor and preserve the legacy of Dr. Sebi. His work has touched the lives of many, and his contributions to the field of natural health are significant. By compiling and presenting his teachings in a structured and comprehensive manner, the book serves as a tribute to his enduring influence. It aims to ensure that his knowledge continues to reach new audiences and inspire future generations to explore the benefits of natural health.

The book also aims to address the misconceptions and skepticism that often surround natural health practices. Dr. Sebi's approach, while unconventional, is rooted in a deep understanding of the body's natural processes and the healing potential of plants. This book will present evidence and testimonials that support the efficacy of his methods, providing a balanced perspective that acknowledges both the strengths and limitations of natural health. By doing so, it aims to foster a more informed and open-minded discussion about alternative approaches to health and wellness.

A practical purpose of the book is to serve as a reference guide that readers can return to time and again. Health is not a static state but a dynamic process that requires continual attention and adjustment. The book will provide practical tools, such as dietary plans, herbal recipes, and detoxification programs, that readers can use to support their health on an ongoing basis. By offering these resources, the book aims to be a valuable companion in the reader's journey towards sustained health and vitality.

In addition to its educational and practical purposes, the book aspires to inspire a deeper connection with nature. Dr. Sebi's teachings emphasize the importance of living in harmony with the natural world, recognizing that our health is intimately connected to the health of the environment. This book will explore this relationship, encouraging readers to adopt a more mindful and eco-conscious approach to their lifestyle. By fostering this connection, the book aims to promote a holistic view of health that encompasses both personal well-being and environmental stewardship.

Finally, the book seeks to create a sense of community among those who follow Dr. Sebi's teachings. Natural health practices often challenge the status quo, and it can be helpful to know that one is not alone on this journey. The book will highlight success stories and testimonials from individuals who have embraced Dr. Sebi's methods and experienced significant health improvements. By sharing these stories, the book aims to build a supportive community of like-minded individuals who can learn from and encourage each other.

In essence, the purpose of this book is to serve as a beacon of knowledge, inspiration, and empowerment. It is a comprehensive guide that illuminates the path to natural health, grounded in the teachings of Dr. Sebi. Whether readers are new to these concepts or seeking to deepen their understanding, the book offers a wealth of information and practical tools to support their journey. It is an invitation to explore the profound benefits of natural health and to embark on a transformative journey towards a healthier, more balanced, and fulfilling life.

Part 1: History and Philosophy of Dr. Sebi

Biography of Dr. Sebi

Life and Education

Alfredo Bowman, known to the world as Dr. Sebi, was born on November 26, 1933, in the humble village of Ilanga in Honduras. His journey into the world of natural healing was neither straightforward nor conventional. Growing up in a rural environment, young Alfredo was deeply influenced by the traditional healing practices he observed. These practices, deeply rooted in the use of natural herbs and plants, planted the seeds of curiosity that would later blossom into his lifelong pursuit of natural health.

From a young age, Dr. Sebi was exposed to the wisdom of his grandmother, Mama Hay, who was a local healer. Mama Hay's vast knowledge of herbs and their medicinal properties left a profound impact on him. He was fascinated by the idea that nature provided all the tools necessary for healing. This early exposure to natural remedies contrasted sharply with the limited access to conventional medicine in his village, shaping his understanding of health and wellness.

Dr. Sebi's formal education was limited, a fact that he often highlighted as both a challenge and a blessing. He struggled with the rigid structure of the traditional education system, which he found stifling and disconnected from the practical knowledge that surrounded him in his everyday life. This disconnect led him to drop out of school at a young age. However, his departure from formal education did not hinder his quest for knowledge. Instead, it propelled him towards a different kind of learning—one that was experiential and deeply connected to his cultural heritage.

As a young man, Dr. Sebi left Honduras and traveled to the United States in search of better opportunities. Settling in New Orleans, he worked various jobs, including that of a steam engineer. His life in America exposed him to a different world, one where the fast-paced, industrial lifestyle starkly contrasted with the natural rhythms he had known in Honduras. This experience broadened his perspective and deepened his resolve to explore natural healing methods.

Despite his lack of formal medical training, Dr. Sebi's insatiable curiosity drove him to study the works of various herbalists, healers, and scientists. He was particularly influenced by the writings of Arnold Ehret, a German healer and proponent of the mucusless diet. Ehret's ideas about the body's natural ability to heal itself through diet and detoxification resonated deeply with Dr. Sebi and became a cornerstone of his own philosophy.

The turning point in Dr. Sebi's life came when he faced a personal health crisis. In his early thirties, he suffered from a range of health issues, including diabetes, asthma, impotency, and obesity. Frustrated by the ineffectiveness of conventional treatments, he decided to turn to the natural remedies he had grown up with. This decision marked the beginning of his self-healing journey and the birth of his commitment to natural health.

Dr. Sebi's personal health transformation was nothing short of miraculous. Through a strict regimen of fasting, herbal treatments, and dietary changes, he managed to overcome his ailments. This profound experience reinforced his belief in the healing power of nature and motivated him to share his knowledge with others. He began to develop a comprehensive system of healing that combined traditional herbal medicine with dietary guidelines aimed at restoring the body's natural alkaline state.

In the 1980s, Dr. Sebi founded the USHA Research Institute in Honduras, named after his mother. The institute became a sanctuary for those seeking alternative treatments for various ailments. Here, he conducted extensive research on the properties of native plants and herbs, developing a range of products designed to cleanse and nourish the body. The success of his treatments attracted people from all over the world, including high-profile individuals who sought his help for their health issues.

Dr. Sebi's approach was holistic, focusing not just on the physical aspects of health but also on emotional and spiritual well-being. He emphasized the importance of diet, detoxification, and the use of natural herbs to create an internal environment that was inhospitable to disease. His philosophy challenged conventional medical paradigms and offered a different perspective on health that resonated with many people.

Throughout his life, Dr. Sebi faced significant opposition from the medical establishment. His lack of formal credentials and the unconventional nature of his methods made him a controversial figure. However, his undeniable results and the testimonies of those he helped provided powerful validation for his work. He remained steadfast in his mission, advocating for natural health and the benefits of an alkaline diet until his passing in 2016.

Dr. Sebi's legacy lives on through the countless lives he touched and the body of work he left behind. His teachings continue to inspire those seeking a natural path to health and wellness. The foundation he laid serves as a guiding light for future generations of healers and health enthusiasts. His life story is a testament to the power of nature and the human spirit's capacity for healing and transformation.

The journey of Dr. Sebi from a small village in Honduras to becoming a renowned natural healer is a remarkable tale of perseverance, curiosity, and unwavering belief in the natural world's healing potential. His life and work underscore the importance of returning to our roots, embracing the wisdom of our ancestors, and trusting in the simple yet profound remedies that nature provides. Dr. Sebi's story is not just a biography; it is an invitation to explore the boundless possibilities of natural health and to reclaim the ancient knowledge that can guide us toward a healthier, more balanced life.

Major Travels and Influences

Dr. Sebi's journey from a small village in Honduras to becoming a renowned figure in natural health was profoundly shaped by his travels and the diverse influences he encountered along the way. Each destination he visited and each culture he immersed himself in contributed to the development of his unique healing philosophy. This blend of experiences provided him with a rich tapestry of knowledge that he wove into his practice, making it both unique and universally resonant.

One of the pivotal moments in Dr. Sebi's life was his decision to leave Honduras and move to the United States. In the vibrant, multicultural environment of New Orleans, he was exposed to a wide array of healing traditions and health practices. This period marked the beginning of his quest to understand the body and its ailments from a holistic perspective. New Orleans, with its rich cultural heritage and blend of African, French, and Caribbean influences, provided fertile ground for his burgeoning interest in herbal medicine and natural healing. During his time in the United States, Dr. Sebi encountered various practitioners of alternative medicine who further broadened his horizons. He learned about the principles of naturopathy, the use of botanical remedies, and the importance of diet in maintaining health. These interactions deepened his understanding and convinced him that natural methods could offer solutions where conventional medicine often fell short. His dissatisfaction with the standard medical treatments he received for his own health issues only fueled his determination to find better alternatives.

Dr. Sebi's travels took him beyond the United States to Mexico, where he found a treasure trove of herbal knowledge. In Mexico, he met indigenous healers who practiced traditional medicine passed down through generations. These healers introduced him to a variety of herbs and plants unknown to him, expanding his repertoire of natural remedies. The indigenous approach to healing, which emphasized harmony with nature and the use of locally sourced plants, resonated deeply with him and reinforced his belief in the efficacy of natural treatments.

Another significant influence on Dr. Sebi was his time spent in Africa. His travels across the continent were not just a return to his ancestral roots but also a profound educational experience. Africa's diverse ecosystems and rich botanical heritage provided him with invaluable insights into the use of medicinal plants. He visited countries like Ghana, where traditional herbal medicine played a central role in health care. The knowledge he gained from African herbalists enriched his understanding of plant-based healing and further validated his own practices. In addition to his travels, Dr. Sebi was heavily influenced by the works of several key figures in the field of natural health. One of the most notable was Arnold Ehret, whose teachings on the mucusless diet and the body's ability to heal itself through proper nutrition had a profound impact on him. Ehret's emphasis on the importance of diet in maintaining health resonated with Dr. Sebi and became a cornerstone of his own philosophy. The idea that an alkaline diet could cleanse the body of toxins and restore health was a revelation that guided much of his subsequent work.

Dr. Sebi's encounters with other health pioneers such as Jethro Kloss, author of "Back to Eden," and Dr. John Christopher, a renowned herbalist, also shaped his understanding of natural healing. These influences helped him to develop a holistic approach that combined the best elements of various traditions. He was not content to merely adopt these teachings; instead, he synthesized them into a cohesive system that reflected his unique insights and experiences. The cumulative impact of Dr. Sebi's travels and the influences he absorbed along the way culminated in the establishment of the USHA Research Institute in Honduras. This center became a hub for his research and a sanctuary for those seeking natural healing. Here, he was able to apply the knowledge he had gathered from around the world, refining his methods and creating a range of herbal products designed to promote health and wellness. The institute also served as a testament to the power of cross-cultural learning and the universal applicability of natural health principles.

Dr. Sebi's journey was characterized by a relentless pursuit of knowledge and a deep respect for the healing traditions of different cultures. His travels not only provided him with practical skills but also enriched his philosophical outlook. He came to view health as a holistic state of being that encompassed physical, emotional, and spiritual dimensions. This perspective was deeply influenced by the holistic approaches he encountered in Africa and the Americas, which emphasized the interconnectedness of all aspects of life.

Throughout his life, Dr. Sebi remained committed to sharing the wisdom he had acquired. He lectured extensively, reaching audiences across the globe and spreading the message of natural health. His teachings emphasized the importance of returning to nature, respecting the body's natural processes, and using food and herbs as medicine. He inspired countless individuals to rethink their approach to health and to explore the benefits of natural remedies.

Dr. Sebi's travels and the diverse influences he absorbed along the way were instrumental in shaping his unique approach to healing. They provided him with a broad and deep understanding of the natural world and its potential to promote health. His experiences across different cultures and environments enriched his knowledge and reinforced his belief in the power of nature. This rich tapestry of influences is reflected in his work, which continues to inspire and guide those seeking a path to wellness through natural means.

In essence, Dr. Sebi's major travels and influences were not just a series of geographical movements but a profound educational journey. They enabled him to gather a wealth of knowledge and to integrate diverse healing traditions into a cohesive and effective system of natural health. His legacy is a testament to the power of learning from different cultures and the enduring value of traditional wisdom in the quest for health and well-being.

Discovery of the Alkaline Diet and Medicinal Herbs

Dr. Sebi's journey to discovering the alkaline diet and the profound medicinal properties of herbs began with his own health crisis. In his early thirties, he was plagued by a range of debilitating ailments including diabetes, asthma, impotency, and obesity. Frustrated by the lack of effective solutions from conventional medicine, he embarked on a personal quest for healing that would ultimately lead him to develop his groundbreaking health philosophy.

Living in the United States, Dr. Sebi was exposed to a diverse range of health practices and dietary philosophies. It was during this time that he encountered the works of Arnold Ehret, a German healer and advocate of the mucusless diet. Ehret's ideas about the body's ability to heal itself through proper nutrition and the elimination of mucus resonated deeply with Dr. Sebi. He was particularly struck by Ehret's assertion that disease is caused by the accumulation of mucus in the body, a concept that would become central to his own teachings.

Inspired by Ehret's work, Dr. Sebi began to experiment with his diet, eliminating foods he believed were contributing to his poor health. He adopted a plant-based diet rich in fresh fruits and vegetables, and noticed significant improvements in his condition. This personal transformation was a revelation, reinforcing his belief in the power of natural foods to heal the body. It also marked the beginning of his commitment to helping others achieve similar results.

As Dr. Sebi delved deeper into his studies, he began to understand the importance of maintaining the body's natural alkaline state. He learned that the pH level of the body is a crucial factor in health, with an alkaline environment promoting well-being and an acidic environment fostering disease. This insight led him to develop the alkaline diet, a nutritional regimen designed to maintain the body's pH balance by focusing on alkaline-forming foods and avoiding acid-forming ones.

The alkaline diet emphasizes the consumption of natural, plant-based foods that are minimally processed. Dr. Sebi identified a range of foods that he believed were particularly beneficial, including leafy greens, fruits, and certain grains and legumes. He also recommended avoiding foods that he considered detrimental to health, such as animal products, processed foods, and those high in starch and sugar. This dietary approach aimed not only to nourish the body but also to detoxify it, removing the accumulated toxins that he believed were the root cause of many diseases.

In addition to the alkaline diet, Dr. Sebi's research led him to explore the medicinal properties of herbs. He traveled extensively, learning from traditional healers and herbalists in Africa, the Americas, and beyond. These experiences deepened his understanding of the healing power of plants and reinforced his belief in the efficacy of natural remedies. He began to develop a range of herbal formulations designed to support the body's natural healing processes.

Dr. Sebi's herbal remedies were based on the principles of African Biomineral Balance, a system he developed that combines traditional African herbal knowledge with modern nutritional science. This system focuses on restoring the body's natural balance through the use of alkaline-forming herbs and foods. He believed that by providing the body with the right nutrients and supporting its detoxification processes, it could heal itself from even the most serious conditions.

One of the key aspects of Dr. Sebi's herbal practice was the use of wildcrafted herbs, which he believed were more potent and effective than their cultivated counterparts. Wildcrafted herbs are those that are harvested from their natural habitats, where they grow without human intervention. Dr. Sebi argued that these herbs retain more of their natural energy and medicinal properties, making them superior to herbs grown in controlled environments.

Among the many herbs Dr. Sebi championed, several stand out for their unique properties and widespread use in his treatments. Sea moss, also known as Irish moss, is rich in minerals and vitamins and is believed to support the immune system and overall health. Burdock root is another important herb in Dr. Sebi's arsenal, known for its detoxifying properties and its ability to cleanse the blood and support liver function. Sarsaparilla, high in iron and other minerals, is used to support blood health and boost energy levels.

Dr. Sebi's approach to herbal medicine was holistic, focusing on the whole person rather than just treating symptoms. He believed that true healing could only occur when the body, mind, and spirit were in harmony. His herbal formulations were designed to address this holistic vision of health, supporting not just physical well-being but also emotional and spiritual balance.

The success of Dr. Sebi's treatments and the transformative impact of his dietary recommendations attracted a diverse following. People from all walks of life sought his guidance, drawn by the promise of natural healing and the testimonials of those who had benefited from his methods. His work garnered attention from high-profile individuals, further elevating his profile and spreading his message to a broader audience.

Despite facing skepticism and opposition from the medical establishment, Dr. Sebi remained steadfast in his commitment to natural health. He continued to refine his methods and share his knowledge, driven by a deep conviction in the power of nature to heal. His dedication to his craft and the tangible results he achieved earned him a loyal following and cemented his legacy as a pioneer in the field of natural health.

Dr. Sebi's discovery of the alkaline diet and medicinal herbs was not just a personal journey but a mission to transform the way we think about health and healing. His work challenges us to reconsider our dietary choices, to embrace the natural world, and to trust in the body's innate ability to heal. Through his teachings, Dr. Sebi has left an indelible mark on the world of natural health, offering a path to wellness that is rooted in simplicity, balance, and the wisdom of nature.

Philosophy of Healing

Basic Principles of the Alkaline Diet

Dr. Sebi's philosophy of healing is deeply rooted in the principles of the alkaline diet. This approach to nutrition is based on the belief that maintaining an alkaline state in the body can prevent and even reverse disease. At the heart of this philosophy is the idea that the foods we consume play a crucial role in determining our body's pH levels. By choosing alkaline-forming foods and avoiding acid-forming ones, we can create an internal environment that supports optimal health.

The alkaline diet is not just a dietary regimen; it is a holistic approach to health that considers the body's need for balance and harmony. Dr. Sebi believed that an acidic internal environment is the breeding ground for disease. This conviction led him to advocate for a diet that is rich in natural, plant-based foods and free from processed, artificial ingredients. According to Dr. Sebi, the key to health lies in returning to nature and consuming foods in their most natural state. Central to the alkaline diet is the consumption of fruits, vegetables, nuts, seeds, and certain grains. These foods are considered alkaline-forming because they help to maintain the body's pH at a slightly alkaline level, which is believed to be ideal for health. For example, leafy greens such as kale and spinach are staples in the alkaline diet due to their high nutrient content and alkalizing effects. Similarly, fruits like lemons and limes, despite their acidic taste, have an alkalizing effect on the body once metabolized.

In contrast, the alkaline diet discourages the consumption of acid-forming foods, which are believed to disrupt the body's pH balance and contribute to the development of disease. These foods include animal products, processed foods, refined sugars, and artificial additives. Dr. Sebi argued that these substances create an acidic environment in the body, leading to inflammation, mucus buildup, and ultimately, disease. By eliminating these foods, individuals can reduce their body's acidic load and promote healing and well-being. One of the fundamental principles of the alkaline diet is its emphasis on whole, unprocessed foods. Dr. Sebi believed that the closer a food is to its natural state, the more beneficial it is for health. This means choosing fresh, organic produce over canned or processed options, and preparing meals from scratch rather than relying on pre-packaged foods. This approach not only ensures that the body receives the maximum nutritional benefit from each food but also minimizes exposure to harmful chemicals and preservatives.

Another key aspect of the alkaline diet is hydration. Dr. Sebi emphasized the importance of drinking natural, alkaline water to support the body's detoxification processes and maintain optimal pH levels. He recommended avoiding tap water, which often contains chlorine and other contaminants, and instead opting for spring water or water that has been naturally alkalized. Proper hydration is essential for flushing out toxins and keeping the body's systems functioning smoothly.

The alkaline diet also includes the use of specific herbs and supplements to support health and healing. Dr. Sebi identified a range of herbs that he believed were particularly effective in promoting an alkaline state and addressing various health issues. These herbs, many of which are indigenous to Central America and Africa, are used to cleanse the blood, support the liver, and boost the immune system. Examples include burdock root, which is known for its detoxifying properties, and sarsaparilla, which is rich in minerals and supports overall vitality. In addition to dietary changes, Dr. Sebi's philosophy of the alkaline diet encourages lifestyle practices that support overall well-being. This includes regular physical activity, sufficient rest, and stress management techniques. By addressing both diet and lifestyle, the alkaline diet takes a comprehensive approach to health that recognizes the interconnectedness of all aspects of life.

The basic principles of the alkaline diet are grounded in the belief that the body is naturally designed to heal itself when given the right conditions. Dr. Sebi argued that many of the chronic diseases plaguing modern society are the result of dietary and lifestyle choices that disrupt the body's natural balance. By adopting an alkaline diet and making other supportive changes, individuals can restore this balance and unlock the body's innate healing potential.

In summary, the alkaline diet is a holistic approach to health that emphasizes the consumption of natural, plant-based foods, proper hydration, and supportive lifestyle practices. Its basic principles are designed to create an internal environment that promotes healing and prevents disease. By understanding and applying these principles, individuals can take control of their health and experience the profound benefits of living in harmony with their body's natural processes. Dr. Sebi's teachings on the alkaline diet continue to inspire and empower those seeking a natural path to wellness, offering a blueprint for a healthier, more balanced life.

The Importance of pH Balance in the Body

Dr. Sebi's philosophy of healing is built on the foundational principle that maintaining an optimal pH balance in the body is crucial for health and vitality. He believed that the body's pH level—whether it is acidic or alkaline—directly influences the state of health or disease. This idea, while simple in its premise, carries profound implications for how we understand and approach wellness.

The human body naturally maintains a slightly alkaline pH, particularly in the blood, which ideally ranges between 7.35 and 7.45. This balance is essential for the proper functioning of metabolic processes, the effectiveness of enzymatic reactions, and the overall health of cells and tissues. Dr. Sebi argued that when this balance is disrupted, particularly by an overly acidic internal environment, the body becomes more susceptible to illness and disease.

An acidic body environment can be caused by various factors, most notably diet and lifestyle choices. Foods that are highly processed, rich in refined sugars, and laden with artificial additives tend to create acidity within the body. Additionally, stress, lack of exercise, and exposure to environmental toxins contribute to this acidic state. Dr. Sebi pointed out that the accumulation of acidity in the body creates a breeding ground for pathogens and contributes to the development of chronic diseases, such as diabetes, hypertension, and arthritis.

Dr. Sebi's advocacy for an alkaline diet stems from this understanding of pH balance. By consuming foods that promote alkalinity, individuals can help counteract the effects of an acidic environment. Alkaline foods—primarily fresh fruits, vegetables, nuts, and seeds—support the body in maintaining its natural pH balance. These foods not only help to neutralize acids but also provide essential nutrients that are crucial for health. For example, leafy greens like kale and spinach are rich in minerals like magnesium and calcium, which are vital for maintaining an alkaline state.

Water is another critical component of pH balance. Dr. Sebi emphasized the importance of drinking alkaline water to help flush out acids and support the body's natural detoxification processes. Unlike tap water, which often contains chemicals that can contribute to acidity, alkaline water helps to maintain the proper pH levels. Hydration is essential not only for pH balance but also for overall health, as it aids in digestion, nutrient absorption, and the elimination of toxins.

The consequences of a disrupted pH balance extend beyond physical health. Dr. Sebi highlighted the interconnectedness of the body, mind, and spirit, suggesting that an acidic environment can also affect mental and emotional well-being. Chronic acidity can lead to fatigue, brain fog, and mood disturbances, which further underscores the importance of maintaining an alkaline state for holistic health.

The significance of pH balance is further underscored by the role it plays in the body's immune function. An alkaline environment supports the immune system by creating conditions that are unfavorable for the growth of harmful bacteria, viruses, and fungi. In contrast, an acidic environment weakens the immune defenses, making the body more vulnerable to infections and illnesses. By adhering to an alkaline diet, individuals can enhance their immune function and improve their resilience against disease.

Another aspect of pH balance that Dr. Sebi emphasized is the body's ability to detoxify. The organs responsible for detoxification, such as the liver and kidneys, function optimally when the body is in an alkaline state. When the body becomes too acidic, these organs are overburdened, and their efficiency in eliminating toxins is compromised. This can lead to the accumulation of harmful substances in the body, further exacerbating health issues. An alkaline diet supports the detoxification process, helping to cleanse the body and maintain internal harmony.

The concept of pH balance also intersects with Dr. Sebi's views on mucus and its role in disease. He believed that excess mucus production is a direct result of an acidic diet and lifestyle. Mucus, which is produced by the body as a protective response to acidity, can become problematic when it accumulates in large amounts. It can obstruct normal bodily functions and provide a breeding ground for bacteria and other pathogens. By maintaining an alkaline state, the production of excess mucus can be minimized, reducing the risk of related health issues.

Dr. Sebi's teachings on pH balance extend to the practical application of this knowledge in everyday life. He encouraged individuals to regularly monitor their pH levels through simple testing methods, such as pH strips, to stay informed about their body's state. This proactive approach allows for timely adjustments in diet and lifestyle to maintain optimal pH balance. Regularly consuming alkaline-forming foods, staying hydrated with alkaline water, and managing stress through techniques like meditation and exercise are all practical steps to achieve and maintain a healthy pH balance.

In summary, the importance of pH balance in the body, as taught by Dr. Sebi, cannot be overstated. It is a cornerstone of his healing philosophy, emphasizing the need to maintain an alkaline internal environment to promote health and prevent disease. By understanding and applying the principles of pH balance, individuals can take significant steps toward achieving holistic wellness. Dr. Sebi's insights into pH balance offer a powerful framework for those seeking to transform their health through natural means, underscoring the profound connection between diet, lifestyle, and overall well-being.

The Concept of Mucus and Disease

A cornerstone of Dr. Sebi's healing philosophy is the concept of mucus and its profound impact on health and disease. According to Dr. Sebi, mucus is the root cause of all disease in the body. This idea diverges significantly from conventional medical theories, which often attribute illness to pathogens, genetics, and lifestyle factors. Dr. Sebi's unique perspective, however, offers a compelling framework for understanding and addressing health issues holistically.

Mucus is a naturally occurring substance in the body, produced by mucous membranes to protect and lubricate various parts of the body, including the respiratory, digestive, and reproductive systems. In normal quantities, mucus serves several vital functions, such as trapping dust and pathogens, aiding in digestion, and facilitating the movement of waste. However, Dr. Sebi argued that an overproduction of mucus, particularly in response to an acidic internal environment, is detrimental to health.

Dr. Sebi believed that when the body is overly acidic, it produces excess mucus as a defense mechanism. This mucus, in turn, can become a breeding ground for bacteria, viruses, and other pathogens, leading to inflammation and disease. For example, excessive mucus in the respiratory system can contribute to conditions such as asthma, bronchitis, and pneumonia. In the digestive system, it can lead to issues like irritable bowel syndrome (IBS), constipation, and bloating. Dr. Sebi's philosophy posits that by reducing mucus production through dietary and lifestyle changes, one can address the underlying cause of many health issues.

Central to Dr. Sebi's approach is the idea that the foods we consume play a critical role in mucus production. He classified foods into two broad categories: mucus-forming and non-mucus-forming. Mucus-forming foods are those that he believed contribute to acidity and excess mucus in the body. These include dairy products, meats, processed foods, and refined sugars. According to Dr. Sebi, these foods should be avoided or minimized to reduce mucus production and maintain a healthy internal environment.

In contrast, non-mucus-forming foods are those that help to alkalize the body and reduce mucus production. These primarily include fresh fruits, vegetables, nuts, seeds, and certain grains. Dr. Sebi advocated for a diet rich in these alkaline-forming foods to support the body's natural detoxification processes and promote overall health. By adopting this dietary approach, individuals can help to clear excess mucus from the body and create conditions that are unfavorable for disease.

Dr. Sebi's emphasis on mucus extends to his views on specific health conditions. He believed that many chronic diseases are manifestations of mucus buildup in various parts of the body. For example, he argued that arthritis is the result of mucus accumulating in the joints, causing inflammation and pain. Similarly, he saw cardiovascular diseases as being linked to mucus buildup in the arteries, which impedes blood flow and leads to heart problems. This perspective offers a unified explanation for a wide range of health issues, emphasizing the importance of addressing the underlying cause rather than merely treating symptoms.

The process of detoxifying the body to remove excess mucus is a key component of Dr. Sebi's healing approach. He recommended periodic fasting and the use of specific herbal remedies to support the body's natural elimination processes. Fasting, according to Dr. Sebi, gives the digestive system a break and allows the body to focus its energy on detoxification and healing. During this time, the body can effectively clear out accumulated mucus and toxins, leading to improved health and vitality.

Herbs also play a crucial role in Dr. Sebi's strategy for reducing mucus and promoting healing. He identified several herbs with powerful detoxifying and alkalizing properties that can help to clear mucus and support the body's natural defenses. For example, burdock root is known for its ability to purify the blood and support liver function, while sarsaparilla is valued for its high mineral content and ability to cleanse the system. These and other herbs are integral to Dr. Sebi's protocols for addressing various health conditions by targeting the root cause: excess mucus.

Dr. Sebi's approach to understanding and treating disease through the lens of mucus production offers a holistic alternative to conventional medical practices. By focusing on the internal environment of the body and the impact of diet and lifestyle on mucus production, he provided a pathway to health that emphasizes prevention and natural healing. This perspective challenges individuals to take a proactive role in their health by making conscious choices that support the body's natural balance and defenses.

One of the most compelling aspects of Dr. Sebi's mucus theory is its simplicity and accessibility. It provides a clear and understandable explanation for why certain foods and habits contribute to disease, and it offers practical steps that anyone can take to improve their health. By reducing or eliminating mucus-forming foods and incorporating more alkaline, non-mucus-forming foods into the diet, individuals can take significant steps toward preventing and reversing disease.

Moreover, Dr. Sebi's focus on mucus highlights the interconnectedness of various bodily systems. It underscores the idea that health is not just about addressing isolated symptoms but about understanding and nurturing the body's holistic balance. This perspective encourages a more integrated approach to health that considers the impact of diet, lifestyle, and environmental factors on overall well-being. Dr. Sebi's concept of mucus and disease represents a radical departure from mainstream medical thought, yet it resonates with many people seeking natural and holistic approaches to health. It emphasizes the body's inherent wisdom and its ability to heal itself when given the right conditions. By adopting Dr. Sebi's principles and focusing on reducing mucus through dietary and lifestyle changes, individuals can take control of their health and experience the transformative benefits of natural healing. In essence, Dr. Sebi's theory of mucus and its role in disease offers a powerful framework for understanding health and illness. It challenges conventional paradigms and provides a pathway to wellness that is grounded in the natural world's wisdom. Through his teachings, Dr. Sebi has inspired countless individuals to rethink their approach to health and to embrace a lifestyle that supports the body's natural balance and healing potential.

Natural Healing and the Use of Herbs

Dr. Sebi's philosophy of natural healing emphasizes the profound relationship between the human body and nature. Central to his teachings is the use of herbs, which he believed to be the most effective means of restoring and maintaining health. Herbs, according to Dr. Sebi, are nature's medicine, providing the essential nutrients and compounds needed to support the body's natural healing processes. This approach to health is rooted in the ancient traditions of herbal medicine, yet it is also informed by modern understandings of nutrition and physiology.

Herbs have been used for centuries across various cultures to treat ailments and promote health. Dr. Sebi's approach draws on this rich tradition, but he also added his unique insights and methods. He believed that the key to natural healing lies in understanding the electrical nature of the human body. The body, he argued, is an electrical organism, and to function optimally, it needs electric foods—foods that are alive and contain high levels of bioavailable nutrients. Herbs, particularly those that are wildcrafted and naturally potent, fit this criterion perfectly. Wildcrafted herbs are those harvested from their natural habitats, where they grow without human intervention. Dr. Sebi favored these herbs because he believed they retained more of their natural energy and medicinal properties compared to commercially farmed herbs. Wildcrafted herbs, according to Dr. Sebi, are more "electric" and thus more effective in restoring the body's natural balance. This perspective underscores his holistic view of health, where the quality and source of the herbs are as important as their specific properties.

Dr. Sebi's approach to herbal medicine is both preventative and curative. He advocated for the regular use of herbs to maintain health and prevent disease, as well as for the treatment of specific conditions. His herbal protocols are designed to cleanse, nourish, and support the body's systems. For example, he often recommended burdock root for its blood-purifying properties, sarsaparilla for its high iron content, and dandelion for its liver-supporting benefits. These herbs are used not just to treat symptoms, but to address the root causes of health issues, supporting the body's natural healing processes.

One of the central tenets of Dr. Sebi's philosophy is detoxification. He believed that the accumulation of toxins in the body is a primary cause of disease. Herbs play a crucial role in detoxification, helping to cleanse the blood, liver, kidneys, and other organs. For example, Dr. Sebi often recommended using herbs such as cascara sagrada and rhubarb root to cleanse the colon, promoting regular bowel movements and the elimination of waste. By supporting the body's natural detoxification processes, these herbs help to remove the buildup of toxins and restore the body to a state of health. In addition to detoxification, Dr. Sebi emphasized the importance of nourishing the body with essential nutrients. Many of the herbs he recommended are rich in vitamins, minerals, and other compounds that support health. For instance, sea moss, also known as Irish moss, is a cornerstone of Dr. Sebi's herbal regimen. This marine plant is packed with minerals, including iodine, calcium, and potassium, which are essential for thyroid function, bone health, and overall cellular function. By incorporating nutrient-dense herbs into the diet, individuals can ensure they are providing their bodies with the raw materials needed for repair and regeneration.

Dr. Sebi's use of herbs extends to his treatment protocols for specific health conditions. He developed detailed herbal regimens for a range of diseases, including diabetes, hypertension, and autoimmune disorders. These protocols often combine multiple herbs to address various aspects of a condition. For example, his approach to treating diabetes might include herbs that help to regulate blood sugar levels, support pancreatic function, and improve overall metabolic health. This multi-faceted approach reflects his understanding of disease as a complex interplay of factors that require a comprehensive treatment strategy. Beyond their physical benefits, Dr. Sebi believed that herbs also support emotional and spiritual health. He viewed the use of herbs as a way to reconnect with nature and restore harmony to the body, mind, and spirit. This holistic perspective is integral to his philosophy of healing, which recognizes that true health encompasses more than just the absence of disease. Herbs, in Dr. Sebi's view, are a means of achieving balance and alignment with the natural world, fostering a deeper sense of well-being.

Dr. Sebi's herbal practices are also characterized by their simplicity and accessibility. He emphasized the use of common, readily available herbs that people could incorporate into their daily routines without the need for expensive or complicated treatments. This approach makes natural healing accessible to a wide audience, empowering individuals to take charge of their health using the resources available to them. Dr. Sebi's teachings encourage people to learn about the herbs growing in their own regions and to use these natural remedies to support their health.

The use of herbs in Dr. Sebi's philosophy is not just about treating disease, but about fostering a lifestyle that supports health and vitality. He encouraged people to view herbal medicine as part of a broader commitment to natural living, which includes a plant-based diet, regular physical activity, and mindful practices such as meditation. This integrative approach reflects his belief in the interconnectedness of all aspects of health and well-being.

Dr. Sebi's legacy in the realm of natural healing and herbal medicine continues to inspire and guide many. His emphasis on the use of herbs as a primary tool for health reflects a deep respect for the wisdom of nature and a commitment to living in harmony with the natural world. By incorporating herbs into their daily lives, individuals can tap into the powerful healing potential of these natural remedies and experience the benefits of holistic health. In summary, Dr. Sebi's approach to natural healing through the use of herbs is a profound testament to the power of nature.

His philosophy integrates traditional herbal wisdom with modern insights, offering a comprehensive framework for achieving and maintaining health. By emphasizing the quality, source, and synergistic use of herbs, Dr. Sebi provided a pathway to wellness that is both deeply rooted in tradition and highly relevant to contemporary health challenges. Through his teachings, he has left a lasting impact on the field of natural healing, inspiring countless individuals to explore the benefits of herbal medicine and embrace a holistic approach to health.

Part 2: Detailed Guide to Herbs

Introduction to Dr. Sebi's Herbs

Definition and Importance of Alkaline Herbs

Dr. Sebi's approach to natural healing is deeply rooted in the use of alkaline herbs, which he considered essential for restoring and maintaining the body's health. Alkaline herbs are those that promote an alkaline environment within the body, helping to balance pH levels and support overall wellness. Dr. Sebi's philosophy emphasizes the importance of these herbs in combating disease, enhancing vitality, and promoting longevity. Understanding the definition and significance of alkaline herbs is fundamental to appreciating the broader context of Dr. Sebi's herbal practices. At its core, the concept of alkaline herbs is based on the idea that the body's optimal state is slightly alkaline. The pH scale, which ranges from 0 to 14, measures how acidic or alkaline a substance is, with 7 being neutral. A pH below 7 is acidic, while a pH above 7 is alkaline. Dr. Sebi believed that maintaining a slightly alkaline pH, particularly in the blood, is crucial for health. He argued that many diseases, including chronic conditions like diabetes, hypertension, and arthritis, stem from an acidic internal environment. Alkaline herbs help to neutralize excess acidity, thus restoring the body's natural balance.

The significance of alkaline herbs extends beyond mere pH adjustment. These herbs are also rich in essential nutrients, including vitamins, minerals, and antioxidants, which support various bodily functions. For example, herbs like burdock root and dandelion are high in iron and other minerals that are vital for blood health and overall energy levels. Sea moss, another key herb in Dr. Sebi's regimen, is packed with iodine, which supports thyroid function and metabolism. By providing these essential nutrients, alkaline herbs not only help to maintain pH balance but also enhance overall nutritional status.

Dr. Sebi's selection of alkaline herbs was influenced by his extensive study of traditional African, Caribbean, and Central American healing practices. He drew on a rich heritage of herbal knowledge, integrating it with his understanding of modern nutrition and biochemistry. This holistic approach ensures that the herbs he recommended are both effective and culturally resonant. For instance, herbs like sarsaparilla, known for its blood-purifying properties, have been used for centuries in various traditional medicine systems. Dr. Sebi's endorsement of such herbs underscores their enduring relevance and efficacy.

In addition to their nutritional benefits, alkaline herbs possess various medicinal properties that support the body's natural healing processes. Many of these herbs are known for their detoxifying effects, helping to cleanse the liver, kidneys, and blood. For example, burdock root is renowned for its ability to remove toxins from the blood and support liver health. Similarly, dandelion root acts as a natural diuretic, promoting kidney function and aiding in the elimination of waste products. By facilitating detoxification, alkaline herbs help to reduce the toxic burden on the body, which can alleviate symptoms and promote recovery from illness.

Another critical aspect of alkaline herbs is their anti-inflammatory properties. Chronic inflammation is a common underlying factor in many diseases, including heart disease, arthritis, and cancer. Alkaline herbs like ginger and turmeric are well-known for their anti-inflammatory effects, which can help to reduce inflammation and support the healing process. These herbs work by inhibiting inflammatory pathways and reducing the production of pro-inflammatory molecules, thereby alleviating pain and swelling. Incorporating such herbs into the diet can provide a natural and effective means of managing inflammation and promoting overall health. The immune-boosting properties of alkaline herbs are also noteworthy. Herbs like echinacea and elderberry have been traditionally used to strengthen the immune system and protect against infections. These herbs contain compounds that enhance immune function, increase the production of white blood cells, and improve the body's ability to fight off pathogens. By supporting the immune system, alkaline herbs help to prevent illness and promote resilience against diseases. This immune-modulating effect is particularly important in maintaining health and preventing the onset of chronic conditions.

Dr. Sebi's emphasis on alkaline herbs is not just about their individual properties but also about their synergistic effects. He believed that combining different herbs could enhance their overall efficacy, providing a more comprehensive approach to healing. For instance, a blend of herbs like burdock root, yellow dock, and dandelion can provide a potent combination of detoxifying, anti-inflammatory, and immune-boosting effects. This holistic approach ensures that the body receives a broad spectrum of benefits, supporting multiple aspects of health simultaneously. Moreover, Dr. Sebi's approach to alkaline herbs is deeply connected to his philosophy of natural living. He advocated for the use of herbs that are grown in their natural environments, free from pesticides and artificial fertilizers. This preference for wildcrafted and organic herbs stems from the belief that such herbs retain more of their natural energy and medicinal properties. Wildcrafted herbs, harvested from their natural habitats, are believed to be more potent and effective than commercially grown varieties. This emphasis on quality and purity is a hallmark of Dr. Sebi's approach, ensuring that the herbs used are as close to their natural state as possible.

The holistic benefits of alkaline herbs extend beyond physical health to encompass mental and emotional well-being. Many of these herbs have adaptogenic properties, helping the body to cope with stress and maintain balance. For example, herbs like ashwagandha and holy basil are known for their ability to reduce stress and improve mood. By supporting the body's stress response, these herbs can help to alleviate anxiety, improve sleep, and enhance overall mental health. This integrative approach to health recognizes the interconnectedness of the body, mind, and spirit, providing a more comprehensive path to wellness.

In summary, alkaline herbs play a central role in Dr. Sebi's philosophy of natural healing. Their ability to promote an alkaline environment in the body, provide essential nutrients, support detoxification, reduce inflammation, boost the immune system, and enhance mental well-being underscores their importance. By integrating these herbs into the diet, individuals can take proactive steps toward restoring and maintaining their health. Dr. Sebi's holistic approach to herbal medicine, grounded in traditional wisdom and modern science, offers a powerful framework for achieving optimal health and vitality.

Differences Between Wildcrafted, Organic, and Commercial Herbs

When exploring the realm of herbal medicine, it's essential to understand the distinctions between wildcrafted, organic, and commercial herbs. These differences are not merely academic but have significant implications for the efficacy, safety, and overall health benefits of the herbs we use. Dr. Sebi's herbal philosophy places a strong emphasis on the quality and sourcing of herbs, advocating for those that are closest to their natural state. This preference underscores the broader principles of his approach to health and wellness, which prioritize natural purity and holistic efficacy.

Wildcrafted herbs are harvested from their natural environments, where they grow without human intervention. These herbs are found in forests, meadows, mountains, and other natural habitats, where they have adapted to their surroundings over centuries. The process of wildcrafting involves collecting these herbs in a sustainable manner that ensures the long-term health of the plant populations and their ecosystems. This method respects the natural growth cycles and habitats of the plants, which is believed to enhance their potency and medicinal properties.

The primary advantage of wildcrafted herbs is their natural purity. Growing in untouched environments, these herbs are free from pesticides, synthetic fertilizers, and other contaminants commonly found in commercial farming. This lack of human interference means that wildcrafted herbs often have higher concentrations of active compounds, making them more effective for medicinal purposes. The belief is that these herbs carry the natural energy and life force of their environments, which can be transferred to those who consume them.

Moreover, the adaptability and resilience of wildcrafted herbs contribute to their effectiveness. Plants that thrive in the wild must endure various environmental stresses, from harsh weather conditions to competition with other plants. This resilience can translate into a greater concentration of beneficial compounds that the plants develop as survival mechanisms. When these herbs are harvested and used for health purposes, they bring these robust properties to the user, potentially offering stronger therapeutic effects.

On the other hand, organic herbs are cultivated under controlled agricultural conditions but without the use of synthetic chemicals. Organic farming practices emphasize sustainability, soil health, and ecological balance. These practices include using natural fertilizers, crop rotation, and biological pest control methods to maintain healthy and productive growing environments. The result is herbs that are free from chemical residues and genetically modified organisms (GMOs), offering a cleaner and more natural product compared to conventional farming methods.

Organic herbs strike a balance between the purity of wildcrafted herbs and the scalability of commercial farming. While they may not have the same level of natural resilience as wildcrafted herbs, they still offer significant health benefits due to their clean cultivation practices. Organic certification ensures that the herbs meet specific standards set by regulatory bodies, providing consumers with assurance about the quality and safety of the products they are using. This certification process includes regular inspections and adherence to strict guidelines, which helps to maintain the integrity of organic herbs.

In contrast, commercial herbs are typically grown in large-scale agricultural operations that prioritize high yields and economic efficiency. These herbs are often exposed to synthetic fertilizers, pesticides, and herbicides, which can leave residues on the plants and impact their overall health benefits. The focus on maximizing production can also lead to practices that deplete soil nutrients and reduce biodiversity, ultimately affecting the quality of the herbs.

Commercially grown herbs may be more accessible and affordable, but they come with trade-offs in terms of purity and potency. The use of synthetic chemicals can introduce harmful substances into the herbs, which may counteract their medicinal benefits. Additionally, the emphasis on quantity over quality can result in herbs with lower concentrations of active compounds, making them less effective for therapeutic purposes. This difference in quality is a significant concern for those who seek to use herbs for health and wellness.

Dr. Sebi's preference for wildcrafted herbs reflects his broader commitment to natural and holistic health practices. He believed that the purity and potency of wildcrafted herbs made them superior for healing purposes. This belief is rooted in the idea that nature provides everything we need for health and that the closer we stay to nature, the better our health outcomes will be. By choosing wildcrafted herbs, Dr. Sebi aimed to harness the full power of nature's pharmacy, ensuring that his treatments were as effective as possible.

Understanding these differences is crucial for making informed choices about herbal products. While wildcrafted herbs offer the highest purity and potency, they may not always be available or practical for everyone. Organic herbs provide a good alternative, offering a balance between natural purity and accessibility. Commercial herbs, while the most widely available, should be approached with caution, especially for those seeking the full therapeutic benefits of herbal medicine.

For those committed to following Dr. Sebi's approach, prioritizing wildcrafted and organic herbs whenever possible is advisable. These options align with his principles of natural purity and holistic health, ensuring that the herbs used in treatments are of the highest quality. However, it is also important to consider sustainability and ethical harvesting practices, particularly with wildcrafted herbs. Ensuring that these plants are collected responsibly helps to protect natural ecosystems and maintain the availability of these valuable resources for future generations.

In summary, the distinctions between wildcrafted, organic, and commercial herbs are significant and impactful. Wildcrafted herbs offer unmatched purity and potency, reflecting the untouched power of nature. Organic herbs provide a balance of purity and practicality, grown under conditions that respect ecological balance and human health. Commercial herbs, while more accessible, often lack the purity and effectiveness of their wildcrafted and organic counterparts. By understanding these differences, individuals can make informed decisions that align with their health goals and the principles of natural healing espoused by Dr. Sebi. This knowledge empowers users to select herbs that not only support their health but also reflect a commitment to natural and sustainable practices.

List of Dr. Sebi's Herbs

Medicinal Properties and Benefits

The medicinal properties and benefits of Dr. Sebi's herbs form the cornerstone of his natural healing approach. These herbs are revered not just for their healing capabilities but also for their ability to support and maintain overall health. Each herb in Dr. Sebi's repertoire is selected for its unique properties, which contribute to the holistic health of the body. Understanding the medicinal properties and benefits of these herbs is essential for anyone looking to incorporate them into their wellness regimen.

Bladderwrack, one of the most celebrated herbs in Dr. Sebi's arsenal, is a type of seaweed known for its high iodine content. This makes it particularly beneficial for thyroid health, as iodine is a crucial element required for the production of thyroid hormones. These hormones regulate metabolism, energy levels, and overall endocrine function. Additionally, bladderwrack is rich in other minerals like calcium, magnesium, and potassium, which support bone health, cardiovascular function, and muscle contractions. Its anti-inflammatory properties also make it useful for reducing pain and swelling in conditions like arthritis.

Burdock root is another key herb that Dr. Sebi frequently recommended. It is renowned for its blood-purifying properties, aiding in the detoxification process by helping the liver and kidneys remove waste from the body. Burdock root is also a powerful antioxidant, which means it helps to protect the body from free radical damage and supports overall cellular health. Its anti-inflammatory and antibacterial properties make it an excellent choice for addressing skin conditions such as eczema, psoriasis, and acne. Moreover, burdock root has been used traditionally to support digestive health, improve appetite, and alleviate gastrointestinal issues.

Sarsaparilla, known for its high iron content, is vital for maintaining healthy blood. Iron is essential for the production of hemoglobin, which transports oxygen throughout the body. This makes sarsaparilla particularly beneficial for individuals with anemia or low energy levels. Additionally, sarsaparilla has diuretic properties, which help to promote kidney health by encouraging the elimination of excess fluids and toxins. Its anti-inflammatory and detoxifying properties further support its use in treating conditions like arthritis and skin disorders. Another notable herb in Dr. Sebi's list is burdock root, which is known for its ability to cleanse the blood and support the lymphatic system. This herb is particularly effective in removing toxins from the bloodstream, thus improving overall health. Burdock root also has diuretic properties, which help to flush out excess water and toxins through urine. Its high antioxidant content protects the body from free radicals, which can damage cells and contribute to chronic diseases. Furthermore, burdock root supports skin health, helping to clear conditions like acne and eczema.

Elderberry is another powerful herb, particularly revered for its immune-boosting properties. Rich in antioxidants, vitamins A and C, and immune-enhancing compounds, elderberry is effective in combating colds, flu, and other respiratory infections. Its antiviral properties make it a popular choice during the cold and flu season, helping to reduce the severity and duration of symptoms. Elderberry also supports cardiovascular health by reducing inflammation and oxidative stress, which are key contributors to heart disease. Nettle leaf is another significant herb recommended by Dr. Sebi. It is a potent anti-inflammatory agent that can help to alleviate symptoms of arthritis and other inflammatory conditions. Nettle leaf is also rich in vitamins and minerals, including iron, calcium, magnesium, and potassium, making it a great supplement for overall health. It supports kidney function by promoting urine production and the elimination of toxins. Additionally, nettle leaf has been used to treat allergies, thanks to its ability to reduce the production of histamines in the body. Chaparral, a lesser-known but equally potent herb, is valued for its detoxifying and anticancer properties. It contains nordihydroguaiaretic acid (NDGA), a powerful antioxidant that helps to inhibit the growth of cancer cells and protect the body from free radical damage. Chaparral is also known for its ability to cleanse the liver, improve digestion, and support the immune system. Its antimicrobial properties make it effective in treating infections and promoting overall health.

Recommended dosages for these herbs can vary depending on the individual's health condition and specific needs. For instance, bladderwrack can be taken as a tea, in capsule form, or as a tincture. A typical dosage might be one to two teaspoons of dried bladderwrack in a cup of hot water, consumed once or twice daily. For burdock root, a common dosage is one to two grams of dried root per day, either as a tea or in capsule form. Sarsaparilla can be taken as a tea or tincture, with a typical dosage being one to two teaspoons of the dried herb in hot water, consumed two to three times daily. The methods of using these herbs are versatile and can be tailored to personal preferences and lifestyles. Infusions, or herbal teas, are a popular method, allowing the active compounds in the herbs to be extracted into hot water. This method is particularly suitable for herbs like nettle leaf, elderberry, and burdock root. Capsules and tablets offer a convenient alternative, especially for those who prefer not to drink herbal teas. Tinctures, which are concentrated herbal extracts made by soaking herbs in alcohol or vinegar, provide a potent and fast-acting option. Topical applications, such as creams or ointments made from herbs like burdock root or chaparral, are effective for treating skin conditions and localized pain.

Incorporating these herbs into daily routines can significantly enhance overall health and well-being. For example, starting the day with an infusion of nettle leaf or burdock root can help to kickstart the detoxification process and provide essential nutrients. Adding bladderwrack or sarsaparilla capsules to a supplement regimen can support thyroid function and blood health. Using elderberry syrup during the cold and flu season can boost the immune system and reduce the severity of symptoms.

Dr. Sebi's emphasis on using herbs as part of a holistic approach to health highlights their role not just in treating specific conditions, but in supporting the body's overall function and resilience. By understanding the medicinal properties, recommended dosages, and methods of use for these key herbs, individuals can harness their full potential and integrate them into a lifestyle that promotes long-term health and vitality. The power of these natural remedies lies in their ability to work synergistically with the body, providing a gentle yet effective means of achieving and maintaining optimal wellness.

Recommended Dosages

Understanding the appropriate dosages for Dr. Sebi's herbs is crucial for maximizing their health benefits while ensuring safety and efficacy. The recommended dosages for these herbs can vary based on factors such as individual health conditions, age, and the specific form of the herb being used. Dr. Sebi emphasized the importance of tailoring dosages to meet individual needs, advocating for a personalized approach to herbal medicine.

Bladderwrack, known for its rich iodine content and benefits for thyroid health, can be taken in various forms, including dried powder, capsules, and tinctures. For dried bladderwrack powder, a typical dosage is about one to two teaspoons per day. This can be mixed with water, juice, or smoothies. When using bladderwrack capsules, it is generally recommended to take 500 to 1000 milligrams per day, divided into two doses. Tinctures are also a popular option; the usual dosage is 2 to 4 milliliters, taken one to three times daily. Adjustments should be made based on individual health needs and responses.

Burdock root, celebrated for its blood-purifying and detoxifying properties, is commonly used in teas, capsules, and tinctures. For burdock root tea, a common dosage is one to two grams of dried root per day, steeped in hot water for 10-15 minutes. This can be consumed up to three times daily. In capsule form, the recommended dosage is typically 300 to 500 milligrams, taken two to three times daily. Tinctures are usually dosed at 2 to 4 milliliters, taken up to three times a day. Consistency is key for achieving the best results with burdock root.

Sarsaparilla, known for its high iron content and blood-purifying abilities, is often taken as a tea, capsule, or tincture. For sarsaparilla tea, the recommended dosage is one to two teaspoons of dried root per cup of hot water, consumed two to three times daily. In capsule form, a typical dosage is 300 to 600 milligrams, taken up to three times per day. Sarsaparilla tinctures are generally dosed at 2 to 4 milliliters, taken up to three times daily. As with other herbs, dosages can be adjusted based on individual needs and health conditions.

Elderberry, renowned for its immune-boosting properties, is commonly used in syrups, capsules, and teas. For elderberry syrup, the standard dosage for adults is one tablespoon taken two to three times daily. During the cold and flu season, this can be increased to four times daily. In capsule form, the recommended dosage is typically 500 to 1000 milligrams, taken once or twice a day. Elderberry tea can be made using one to two teaspoons of dried berries per cup of hot water, consumed two to three times daily.

Nettle leaf, valued for its anti-inflammatory and nutrient-rich properties, can be used in teas, capsules, and tinctures. For nettle leaf tea, a common dosage is one to two teaspoons of dried leaves per cup of hot water, consumed two to three times daily. In capsule form, the typical dosage is 300 to 500 milligrams, taken two to three times per day. Nettle leaf tinctures are usually dosed at 2 to 5 milliliters, taken up to three times a day. Nettle can be particularly beneficial when taken consistently over time to support overall health and vitality.

Chaparral, known for its detoxifying and anticancer properties, is typically used in teas and tinctures. For chaparral tea, the recommended dosage is one teaspoon of dried herb per cup of hot water, consumed once or twice daily. In tincture form, the usual dosage is 1 to 3 milliliters, taken two to three times daily. Given its potency, it is important to use chaparral with caution and to consult with a healthcare provider before starting regular use, especially for individuals with preexisting health conditions. Each of these herbs offers unique benefits and can be used in various forms to suit individual preferences and health needs. Infusions, or herbal teas, are a popular and accessible method of using these herbs, allowing their active compounds to be extracted into hot water. This method is particularly suitable for herbs like nettle leaf, elderberry, and burdock root, providing a soothing and enjoyable way to consume these medicinal plants.

Capsules and tablets offer a convenient alternative, especially for those who may not enjoy the taste of herbal teas or who need a portable option. These forms ensure consistent dosages and are easy to incorporate into daily routines. Tinctures, which are concentrated herbal extracts made by soaking herbs in alcohol or vinegar, provide a potent and fast-acting option. They are especially useful for those who need quick relief or prefer a more concentrated form of the herb.

Topical applications, such as creams, ointments, and poultices, can be particularly effective for treating localized conditions like skin irritations, wounds, and joint pain. Herbs like burdock root and chaparral can be made into poultices to apply directly to the skin, providing targeted relief and supporting the healing process. These methods allow the active compounds in the herbs to be absorbed directly through the skin, offering a different mode of action compared to internal use. The versatility of these herbs means they can be tailored to individual needs and preferences, making it easier to integrate them into daily health routines. For example, starting the day with an infusion of nettle leaf or burdock root can help kickstart the detoxification process and provide essential nutrients. Adding bladderwrack or sarsaparilla capsules to a supplement regimen can support thyroid function and blood health. Using elderberry syrup during the cold and flu season can boost the immune system and reduce the severity of symptoms.

Dr. Sebi's emphasis on the proper use and dosage of herbs highlights the importance of knowledge and care in herbal medicine. By understanding the recommended dosages and methods of use, individuals can maximize the benefits of these powerful plants while minimizing potential risks. It is always advisable to start with lower dosages and gradually increase as needed, paying close attention to how the body responds.

Moreover, consulting with a healthcare provider or a knowledgeable herbalist can provide additional guidance and ensure that the use of these herbs is safe and appropriate for individual health conditions. This personalized approach to herbal medicine aligns with Dr. Sebi's philosophy of holistic health, which considers the unique needs and circumstances of each person.

Incorporating these herbs into daily routines can significantly enhance overall health and well-being. Consistency and mindfulness in their use are key to achieving the best results. By following the recommended dosages and methods of use, individuals can harness the full potential of Dr. Sebi's herbs and experience the transformative benefits of natural healing.

Methods of Use

Understanding how to properly use Dr. Sebi's herbs is essential for unlocking their full potential and ensuring they contribute effectively to health and wellness. The methods of use for these herbs vary depending on the form in which they are consumed, including infusions, capsules, and topical applications. Each method has its unique advantages, and choosing the right one depends on personal preference, specific health needs, and the type of herb being used.

Infusions, or herbal teas, are one of the most traditional and accessible methods of using herbs. This method involves steeping dried herbs in hot water to extract their medicinal properties. Infusions are particularly suitable for herbs like nettle leaf, elderberry, and burdock root. To prepare an infusion, begin by boiling water and allowing it to cool slightly. Place one to two teaspoons of the dried herb in a tea infuser or directly into a cup, and pour the hot water over the herbs. Cover the cup to retain the heat and let it steep for about 10-15 minutes. Strain the herbs if necessary, and the infusion is ready to drink. This method allows the active compounds to be easily absorbed and enjoyed in a soothing beverage.

Capsules and tablets offer a convenient and straightforward alternative, especially for those who may not enjoy the taste of herbal teas or who need a portable option. These forms ensure consistent dosages and are easy to incorporate into daily routines. For example, bladderwrack capsules can be taken with water during meals to support thyroid health and provide essential minerals. Burdock root capsules are another option for those seeking to cleanse their blood and support liver function without the need to prepare an infusion.

Tinctures, which are concentrated herbal extracts made by soaking herbs in alcohol or vinegar, provide a potent and fast-acting option. Tinctures are especially useful for those who need quick relief or prefer a more concentrated form of the herb. To use a tincture, measure the recommended dosage using a dropper and place the drops under the tongue or mix them with a small amount of water or juice. This method allows the active compounds to enter the bloodstream quickly, providing rapid therapeutic effects. For instance, sarsaparilla tincture can be used to boost iron levels and support overall energy.

Topical applications, such as creams, ointments, and poultices, are particularly effective for treating localized conditions like skin irritations, wounds, and joint pain. Herbs like burdock root and chaparral can be made into poultices to apply directly to the skin, providing targeted relief and supporting the healing process. To make a poultice, combine the dried herb with a small amount of hot water to create a paste. Spread the paste onto a clean cloth and apply it to the affected area, securing it with a bandage if necessary. Leave the poultice in place for about 20-30 minutes, then remove it and rinse the area with warm water. This method allows the active compounds to be absorbed directly through the skin, offering a different mode of action compared to internal use.

For those interested in making their own herbal capsules, start by grinding the dried herbs into a fine powder using a mortar and pestle or an electric grinder. Fill empty gelatin or vegetable capsules with the powdered herb using a capsule machine or manually. This DIY approach allows for customization of dosages and combinations of different herbs. Homemade capsules can be stored in a cool, dry place and taken as needed to support various health goals.

Another effective method is the use of herbal baths. Adding herbs to a warm bath can provide therapeutic benefits through both skin absorption and inhalation of aromatic compounds. To prepare an herbal bath, fill a muslin bag or cheesecloth with the desired herbs and tie it securely. Place the bag in the bathtub as it fills with warm water, allowing the herbs to steep and release their properties. Alternatively, prepare a strong infusion by steeping the herbs in hot water, then strain and add the liquid to the bathwater. Soak in the herbal bath for 20-30 minutes to relax, soothe sore muscles, and nourish the skin.

Herbal oils are another versatile option for using Dr. Sebi's herbs. Infusing herbs in carrier oils like olive, coconut, or almond oil allows for easy application and absorption through the skin. To make herbal oil, fill a glass jar with dried herbs and cover them with the carrier oil. Seal the jar and place it in a sunny window for two to six weeks, shaking it gently every few days. After the infusion period, strain the oil through a cheesecloth or fine mesh strainer, and store it in a dark, cool place. Herbal oils can be used for massages, added to lotions, or applied directly to the skin for various benefits.

Herbal syrups combine the therapeutic properties of herbs with the sweetness of natural sweeteners like honey or maple syrup, making them palatable and enjoyable. Elderberry syrup is a popular example, known for its immune-boosting effects. To make elderberry syrup, simmer dried elderberries with water and spices like cinnamon and cloves for about 30-45 minutes. Strain the liquid, discard the solids, and stir in honey while the liquid is still warm. Store the syrup in the refrigerator and take it by the tablespoon daily, especially during the cold and flu season, to support immune health.

Herbal lozenges are another creative way to incorporate Dr. Sebi's herbs into your routine, particularly for soothing sore throats and respiratory issues. To make herbal lozenges, combine powdered herbs with a natural binder like honey or glycerin to form a thick paste. Roll the paste into small balls and flatten them into lozenge shapes. Allow the lozenges to dry and harden, then store them in an airtight container. These lozenges can be sucked on throughout the day to relieve symptoms and provide continuous benefits.

Incorporating these methods into daily routines can significantly enhance overall health and well-being. Consistency and mindfulness in their use are key to achieving the best results. For example, starting the day with an infusion of nettle leaf or burdock root can help kickstart the detoxification process and provide essential nutrients. Adding bladderwrack or sarsaparilla capsules to a supplement regimen can support thyroid function and blood health. Using elderberry syrup during the cold and flu season can boost the immune system and reduce the severity of symptoms.

Dr. Sebi's emphasis on the proper use and dosage of herbs highlights the importance of knowledge and care in herbal medicine. By understanding the recommended dosages and methods of use, individuals can maximize the benefits of these powerful plants while minimizing potential risks. It is always advisable to start with lower dosages and gradually increase as needed, paying close attention to how the body responds. Moreover, consulting with a healthcare provider or a knowledgeable herbalist can provide additional guidance and ensure that the use of these herbs is safe and appropriate for individual health conditions. This personalized approach to herbal medicine aligns with Dr. Sebi's philosophy of holistic health, which considers the unique needs and circumstances of each person.

By integrating these various methods of use into daily health routines, individuals can fully harness the therapeutic potential of Dr. Sebi's herbs, achieving a balanced and natural approach to wellness. Whether through infusions, capsules, tinctures, topical applications, or other creative methods, the key is to maintain a consistent and mindful practice that supports the body's natural healing processes. This comprehensive approach to using herbs not only promotes physical health but also fosters a deeper connection to nature and a more holistic sense of well-being.

Key Herbs

Dr. Sebi's herbal practice includes a variety of powerful herbs, each with unique properties and benefits. These key herbs are central to his natural healing philosophy, offering a range of therapeutic effects that support overall health and address specific ailments. Understanding these herbs can provide valuable insights into their roles in promoting wellness and vitality.

Bladderwrack, a type of seaweed, is highly valued for its rich iodine content. Iodine is essential for thyroid health, helping to regulate metabolism and support endocrine function. Bladderwrack also contains a variety of other minerals, including calcium, magnesium, and potassium, which are vital for bone health, muscle function, and cardiovascular well-being. Additionally, bladderwrack has anti-inflammatory properties, making it beneficial for conditions like arthritis and joint pain. It can be taken as a tea, in capsules, or as a tincture. For a tea, steep one to two teaspoons of dried bladderwrack in hot water for 10-15 minutes. For capsules, the recommended dosage is typically 500 to 1000 milligrams per day, and for tinctures, 2 to 4 milliliters taken one to three times daily.

Burdock root is renowned for its detoxifying properties. It supports liver and kidney function by helping to remove toxins from the body. Burdock root is also a powerful antioxidant, protecting cells from damage caused by free radicals. Its anti-inflammatory and antibacterial properties make it effective in treating skin conditions like acne, eczema, and psoriasis. Burdock root can be used as a tea, in capsules, or as a tincture. To prepare a tea, steep one to two grams of dried burdock root in hot water for 10-15 minutes. For capsules, the recommended dosage is 300 to 500 milligrams, taken two to three times daily. For tinctures, the usual dosage is 2 to 4 milliliters, taken up to three times per day.

Sarsaparilla is another key herb known for its high iron content, which is crucial for maintaining healthy blood and preventing anemia. Sarsaparilla also has diuretic properties, promoting kidney health by encouraging the elimination of excess fluids and toxins. Its anti-inflammatory and detoxifying effects make it useful for treating conditions like arthritis and skin disorders. Sarsaparilla can be consumed as a tea, in capsules, or as a tincture. For a tea, steep one to two teaspoons of dried sarsaparilla root in hot water for 10-15 minutes. For capsules, the recommended dosage is 300 to 600 milligrams, taken up to three times daily. For tinctures, the dosage is typically 2 to 4 milliliters, taken two to three times daily.

Sea moss, also known as Irish moss, is a nutrient powerhouse. It is rich in minerals like iodine, calcium, magnesium, and potassium, which support various bodily functions, including thyroid health, bone health, and overall cellular function. Sea moss also has mucilaginous properties, which means it helps to soothe and protect the mucous membranes, making it beneficial for respiratory and digestive health. Sea moss can be consumed in gel form, capsules, or as a tea. To make sea moss gel, soak the dried sea moss in water for several hours, then blend it with fresh water until smooth. The gel can be added to smoothies, soups, or taken by the spoonful. For capsules, the recommended dosage is typically 500 to 1000 milligrams per day.

Yellow dock is a powerful herb known for its blood-purifying and detoxifying properties. It supports liver function and helps to cleanse the blood by promoting the elimination of toxins. Yellow dock is also high in iron and other minerals, making it beneficial for addressing anemia and boosting energy levels. Its laxative properties can help to relieve constipation and promote healthy digestion. Yellow dock can be used as a tea, in capsules, or as a tincture. To prepare a tea, steep one teaspoon of dried yellow dock root in hot water for 10-15 minutes. For capsules, the recommended dosage is 300 to 500 milligrams, taken two to three times daily. For tinctures, the dosage is typically 2 to 4 milliliters, taken up to three times daily.

Dandelion root is celebrated for its diuretic properties, which help to promote kidney health and support detoxification. It also aids in liver function, helping to eliminate toxins from the body. Dandelion root is high in vitamins and minerals, including vitamins A, C, and K, as well as calcium, potassium, and magnesium. These nutrients support overall health and well-being. Dandelion root can be consumed as a tea, in capsules, or as a tincture. To prepare a tea, steep one to two teaspoons of dried dandelion root in hot water for 10-15 minutes. For capsules, the recommended dosage is 300 to 500 milligrams, taken two to three times daily. For tinctures, the dosage is typically 2 to 4 milliliters, taken up to three times daily.

Nettle leaf is another significant herb in Dr. Sebi's repertoire, known for its anti-inflammatory and nutrient-rich properties. It is high in vitamins A, C, K, and several B vitamins, as well as minerals like iron, calcium, magnesium, and potassium. Nettle leaf supports kidney function by promoting urine production and the elimination of toxins. It also has antihistamine properties, making it useful for treating allergies. Nettle leaf can be used as a tea, in capsules, or as a tincture. To prepare a tea, steep one to two teaspoons of dried nettle leaf in hot water for 10-15 minutes. For capsules, the recommended dosage is 300 to 500 milligrams, taken two to three times daily. For tinctures, the dosage is typically 2 to 5 milliliters, taken up to three times daily.

Chaparral is known for its detoxifying and anticancer properties. It contains nordihydroguaiaretic acid (NDGA), a powerful antioxidant that helps to inhibit the growth of cancer cells and protect the body from free radical damage. Chaparral is also known for its ability to cleanse the liver, improve digestion, and support the immune system. Its antimicrobial properties make it effective in treating infections and promoting overall health. Chaparral can be used as a tea or tincture. To prepare a tea, steep one teaspoon of dried chaparral in hot water for 10-15 minutes. For tinctures, the usual dosage is 1 to 3 milliliters, taken two to three times daily.

Each of these herbs offers unique benefits and can be used in various forms to suit individual preferences and health needs. Infusions, or herbal teas, allow the active compounds in the herbs to be extracted into hot water, providing a soothing and enjoyable way to consume these medicinal plants. Capsules and tablets offer a convenient alternative, especially for those who may not enjoy the taste of herbal teas or who need a portable option. Tinctures provide a potent and fast-acting option, delivering concentrated herbal extracts directly into the bloodstream for rapid therapeutic effects. Topical applications, such as creams, ointments, and poultices, are effective for treating localized conditions like skin irritations, wounds, and joint pain. Incorporating these herbs into daily routines can significantly enhance overall health and well-being. Consistency and mindfulness in their use are key to achieving the best results. For example, starting the day with an infusion of nettle leaf or burdock root can help kickstart the detoxification process and provide essential nutrients. Adding bladderwrack or sarsaparilla capsules to a supplement regimen can support thyroid function and blood health. Using elderberry syrup during the cold and flu season can boost the immune system and reduce the severity of symptoms.

Dr. Sebi's emphasis on the proper use and dosage of herbs highlights the importance of knowledge and care in herbal medicine. By understanding the medicinal properties, recommended dosages, and methods of use for these key herbs, individuals can maximize their health benefits and support overall wellness. This holistic approach to using herbs not only promotes physical health but also fosters a deeper connection to nature and a more balanced, natural lifestyle.

Sourcing and Storage of Herbs

Where to Find the Herbs

Finding high-quality herbs is a critical step in ensuring their efficacy and safety. The first consideration is the source. Herbs can be found in various places, including local markets, health food stores, online retailers, and, for the more adventurous, directly from nature. Each source has its advantages and potential drawbacks, which must be carefully considered to ensure you are getting the best product.

Local farmers' markets and health food stores often carry a selection of fresh and dried herbs. These venues typically source their products from local or regional growers, which can mean fresher herbs and a lower environmental impact due to reduced transportation distances. Shopping locally also allows you to ask vendors directly about their farming practices, ensuring that the herbs are grown without synthetic pesticides or fertilizers. This can provide a higher level of confidence in the quality and purity of the herbs.

Online retailers offer a vast selection of herbs from around the world, providing access to rare and exotic varieties that may not be available locally. When purchasing herbs online, it's essential to buy from reputable sources. Look for companies that provide detailed information about their sourcing practices, including whether the herbs are organic, wildcrafted, or ethically harvested. Reading customer reviews and checking for third-party certifications can also help ensure the quality of the products. Trusted online sources often provide comprehensive product information, including lab testing results for contaminants and potency.

For those who prefer a hands-on approach, foraging for wild herbs can be a rewarding experience. This method allows you to connect directly with nature and source herbs in their most natural state. However, foraging requires a good understanding of plant identification and local regulations, as some herbs can be easily confused with toxic look-alikes, and foraging may be restricted in certain areas to protect ecosystems. It's crucial to forage responsibly, taking only what you need and leaving enough for the plant population to remain healthy and sustainable.

Growing your own herbs is another excellent option for ensuring a steady supply of high-quality medicinal plants. Home gardening allows for complete control over the growing conditions, including soil quality, water, and the absence of harmful chemicals. Many medicinal herbs are easy to grow and thrive in various climates. Starting a home herb garden can be as simple as planting seeds or seedlings in pots or garden beds and providing them with proper care. This method not only ensures a fresh supply of herbs but also fosters a deeper connection to the plants and their life cycles.

How to Harvest and Store Herbs

Harvesting herbs at the right time is crucial for maximizing their medicinal properties. The timing of the harvest depends on the specific plant and the part being used, whether it's the leaves, flowers, roots, or seeds. Generally, leaves and flowers are best harvested in the morning after the dew has evaporated but before the heat of the day. This timing helps preserve the essential oils, which are responsible for much of the herb's therapeutic properties. Roots are typically harvested in the fall when the plant's energy is concentrated below ground, and seeds are collected once they are fully mature and dry.

To harvest herbs, use clean, sharp scissors or pruners to avoid damaging the plant. Cut above a leaf node or bud to encourage new growth and ensure the plant continues to thrive. For leaves and flowers, gather them in small bunches and tie them with string, then hang them upside down in a cool, dark, and well-ventilated area to dry. This method helps preserve the color, flavor, and medicinal properties. For roots, wash them thoroughly to remove soil, then chop them into small pieces and dry them in a similar manner. Seeds should be collected and spread out on a flat surface in a well-ventilated area to dry completely before storing.

Proper storage of dried herbs is essential to maintain their potency and extend their shelf life. Once dried, store herbs in airtight containers, such as glass jars, to protect them from air, moisture, and light. Label the containers with the name of the herb and the date of harvest to keep track of their freshness. Store the containers in a cool, dark place, such as a pantry or cupboard, away from direct sunlight and heat sources. When stored correctly, most dried herbs will retain their medicinal properties for up to a year.

Preparation and Storage for Long-Term Use

Preparing herbs for long-term use involves several methods, each suited to different types of herbs and intended uses. Infusions and decoctions are common ways to extract the medicinal properties of herbs for immediate use, but for long-term storage, tinctures, herbal oils, and salves are more appropriate.

Tinctures are concentrated herbal extracts made by soaking herbs in alcohol or vinegar. To make a tincture, fill a glass jar with fresh or dried herbs, then cover them with high-proof alcohol, such as vodka, or apple cider vinegar. Seal the jar tightly and store it in a cool, dark place for four to six weeks, shaking it gently every few days. After the extraction period, strain the liquid through a fine mesh strainer or cheesecloth into a clean jar, and label it with the herb name and date. Tinctures have a long shelf life, often lasting several years if stored properly.

Herbal oils are made by infusing herbs in carrier oils, such as olive, coconut, or almond oil. To prepare an herbal oil, place dried herbs in a glass jar and cover them with the carrier oil. Seal the jar and place it in a sunny window for two to six weeks, shaking it gently every few days. After the infusion period, strain the oil through a cheesecloth or fine mesh strainer into a clean container. Store the herbal oil in a cool, dark place, and it will keep for several months to a year. Herbal oils can be used for massages, added to lotions, or applied directly to the skin for various therapeutic effects.

Salves are made by combining herbal oils with beeswax to create a semi-solid, easy-to-apply ointment. To make a salve, gently heat the herbal oil in a double boiler, then add grated beeswax and stir until melted and thoroughly combined. Pour the mixture into small jars or tins and allow it to cool and solidify. Label the containers with the herb name and date. Salves are excellent for treating skin conditions, providing localized relief from pain and inflammation, and supporting overall skin health.

Another method for long-term storage is drying and powdering herbs. Once herbs are thoroughly dried, they can be ground into a fine powder using a mortar and pestle or an electric grinder. Store the powdered herbs in airtight containers, away from light and moisture. This method is particularly useful for herbs that are used in capsules or added to food and drinks for their medicinal properties.

For those who prefer convenience, encapsulating powdered herbs is an effective way to store and consume them. You can purchase empty gelatin or vegetable capsules and a capsule-filling machine to make your own herbal supplements. This method allows you to customize dosages and create blends of different herbs tailored to your specific health needs. Store the filled capsules in airtight containers, labeled with the herb names and dates, and keep them in a cool, dark place to maintain their potency. By understanding where to find, how to harvest, and how to store herbs properly, you can ensure that you are getting the most out of these natural remedies. Whether sourcing from local markets, foraging, or growing your own, the quality and care taken in these processes will significantly impact the effectiveness of the herbs in promoting health and wellness. Proper storage and preparation techniques further enhance the longevity and potency of these valuable plants, allowing you to maintain a natural and holistic approach to health throughout the year.

Part 3: Diet Plans and Recipes

Principles of the Alkaline Diet

Principles of the Alkaline Diet

The alkaline diet, rooted in the work of Dr. Sebi, proposes a unique perspective on nutrition and health. At its core, it suggests that maintaining the body's pH balance through dietary choices can prevent and even reverse diseases. This approach hinges on the consumption of alkaline foods while avoiding those that produce acid. Let's delve into the specifics of what foods are permitted and which are forbidden, and explore the fundamental benefits of adhering to an alkaline diet.

Understanding the distinction between alkaline and acidic foods is essential for anyone looking to adopt this dietary regimen. Alkaline foods, often referred to as "electric foods" by Dr. Sebi, are those that help maintain the body's natural pH balance, which ideally hovers around 7.4 on the pH scale. These foods typically include a variety of fruits, vegetables, nuts, and grains. Forbidden foods, on the other hand, are those that create acid in the body and can disrupt this delicate balance, leading to a host of health issues.

Let's start with the foods that are encouraged on the alkaline diet. Fresh fruits and vegetables are the cornerstones of this dietary plan. Leafy greens such as kale, spinach, and Swiss chard are particularly emphasized due to their high alkaline content. Other vegetables like cucumbers, bell peppers, and zucchini also play a crucial role. Fruits such as apples, bananas, berries, and melons are not only alkaline but also packed with essential vitamins and antioxidants.

In addition to fruits and vegetables, certain nuts and seeds are considered beneficial. Almonds, flaxseeds, and chia seeds, for instance, provide essential fatty acids and proteins without disrupting the body's pH balance. Grains such as quinoa, millet, and spelt are preferred over more common grains like wheat and rice, which are more acid-forming. Conversely, the alkaline diet places a significant emphasis on avoiding foods that are acid-producing. Processed foods are at the top of this list, including anything that contains refined sugars, artificial additives, or preservatives. These foods not only create an acidic environment in the body but also contribute to inflammation and other health issues. Dairy products are also restricted on the alkaline diet. While many people consume milk, cheese, and yogurt as part of their daily diet, these foods can lead to mucus production and acidification in the body. Dr. Sebi's approach advocates for plant-based alternatives such as almond milk or coconut yogurt.

Animal proteins, including meat, poultry, and fish, are another category of foods to avoid. These proteins, though rich in essential amino acids, are highly acid-forming and can put a strain on the body's natural pH balance. Instead, plant-based protein sources such as lentils, chickpeas, and various nuts are recommended.

Grains such as wheat, rice, and oats are typically staples in many diets, but they are considered acid-forming and are thus restricted. In place of these, the alkaline diet promotes the use of quinoa, amaranth, and spelt, which are less likely to disrupt the body's pH levels.

The benefits of adhering to an alkaline diet are numerous and compelling. One of the most significant advantages is the potential for disease prevention and improved overall health. An alkaline environment in the body can help reduce inflammation, which is a common underlying factor in many chronic diseases, including arthritis, heart disease, and even cancer. By consuming a diet rich in alkaline foods, individuals may experience reduced symptoms of these conditions and an overall enhancement in their quality of life.

Energy levels are another area where the alkaline diet can have a profound impact. Many people who switch to an alkaline diet report increased energy and vitality. This boost in energy can be attributed to the body operating more efficiently in a balanced pH environment. Acidic foods can lead to fatigue and sluggishness, whereas alkaline foods support optimal cellular function and energy production.

Weight management is another benefit often associated with the alkaline diet. Because the diet focuses on whole, unprocessed foods, it naturally reduces the intake of high-calorie, low-nutrient foods that contribute to weight gain. Additionally, an alkaline diet can help balance hormones and improve metabolism, further supporting healthy weight loss and maintenance.

Digestive health is also positively influenced by an alkaline diet. Many alkaline foods are high in fiber, which promotes healthy digestion and regular bowel movements. Furthermore, a balanced pH can help maintain the integrity of the gut lining and support a healthy microbiome, both of which are crucial for optimal digestive function.

Skin health is yet another area where the alkaline diet shines. The high intake of fruits and vegetables provides essential vitamins and antioxidants that promote healthy, glowing skin. Moreover, reducing the intake of acidic foods can help minimize skin conditions such as acne, eczema, and psoriasis.

Mental clarity and mood stabilization are additional benefits. The reduction in inflammation and the improvement in overall health can have a positive effect on mental well-being. Many followers of the alkaline diet report better focus, reduced anxiety, and a more stable mood.

In adopting the alkaline diet, individuals are encouraged to make gradual changes rather than drastic shifts. This approach allows the body to adjust to the new way of eating and helps ensure long-term adherence to the diet. Starting with small steps, such as incorporating more fruits and vegetables into daily meals and slowly reducing the intake of acidic foods, can make the transition smoother and more sustainable.

The alkaline diet, as promoted by Dr. Sebi, is more than just a dietary regimen; it is a lifestyle that emphasizes the importance of natural, unprocessed foods for maintaining health and preventing disease. By focusing on foods that support the body's natural pH balance and avoiding those that disrupt it, individuals can achieve significant improvements in their overall health and well-being. Whether it's through enhanced energy levels, better weight management, or improved digestive health, the benefits of the alkaline diet are both profound and far-reaching.

Benefits of the Alkaline Diet

The alkaline diet, as championed by Dr. Sebi, offers a transformative approach to health and wellness that extends far beyond simple nutrition. Its benefits, rooted in the intricate balance of the body's pH levels, are profound and multifaceted. By embracing an alkaline diet, individuals can experience a cascade of positive changes, impacting everything from cellular function to overall vitality.

One of the most compelling benefits of the alkaline diet is its potential to reduce inflammation. Chronic inflammation is a silent contributor to a host of debilitating conditions, including heart disease, arthritis, and autoimmune disorders. The foods emphasized in the alkaline diet—fresh fruits, vegetables, nuts, and seeds—are rich in antioxidants and phytochemicals that combat oxidative stress, a key driver of inflammation. By minimizing acidic foods that can trigger inflammatory responses, the diet helps create an internal environment where inflammation is less likely to thrive, fostering overall wellness.

Another significant advantage is the enhancement of energy levels. Many who adopt the alkaline diet report a noticeable increase in their energy and stamina. This surge can be attributed to the diet's emphasis on nutrient-dense foods that provide sustained energy. Alkaline foods facilitate efficient metabolic processes, ensuring that cells have the necessary nutrients to function optimally. When the body isn't bogged down by the need to neutralize excessive acidity, energy is freed up for more vital functions, leading to a vibrant, energized feeling throughout the day.

Weight management is also a prominent benefit. The alkaline diet naturally curtails the intake of processed, high-sugar foods that contribute to weight gain. Instead, it promotes whole, plant-based foods that are lower in calories and higher in essential nutrients. This shift not only supports healthy weight loss but also helps in maintaining an ideal weight. Moreover, the diet's focus on high-fiber foods enhances satiety, reducing the likelihood of overeating and snacking between meals. Digestive health is profoundly impacted by an alkaline diet. The high fiber content of fruits, vegetables, and whole grains supports regular bowel movements and the maintenance of a healthy gut microbiome. A balanced gut flora is crucial for optimal digestion and the prevention of conditions like constipation, bloating, and irritable bowel syndrome. Additionally, the alkaline diet can help repair and maintain the integrity of the gut lining, reducing the risk of leaky gut syndrome and other gastrointestinal disorders.

The benefits of the alkaline diet extend to cardiovascular health as well. By prioritizing foods that are low in saturated fats and cholesterol, the diet helps reduce the risk of atherosclerosis, hypertension, and other heart-related issues. The abundance of potassium-rich foods like bananas, avocados, and leafy greens supports heart health by helping to regulate blood pressure. Furthermore, the anti-inflammatory properties of the diet play a crucial role in protecting the cardiovascular system from damage.

Skin health is another area where the alkaline diet proves its worth. The nutrient-rich foods emphasized in this diet provide essential vitamins and minerals that promote healthy, glowing skin. Vitamin C from fruits like oranges and strawberries aids in collagen production, while the antioxidants in leafy greens and nuts protect the skin from damage caused by free radicals. Many followers of the alkaline diet report clearer, more radiant skin, with a reduction in issues such as acne and eczema.

Mental clarity and emotional well-being are also enhanced by the alkaline diet. The brain requires a constant supply of nutrients to function optimally, and the alkaline diet provides these in abundance. Foods rich in omega-3 fatty acids, such as flaxseeds and walnuts, support cognitive function and reduce the risk of mental decline. Additionally, the reduction in inflammation and oxidative stress benefits brain health, leading to improved focus, memory, and overall mental performance. Emotional well-being is bolstered by stable blood sugar levels and the absence of artificial additives and preservatives, which can negatively impact mood.

The immune system reaps significant benefits from an alkaline diet. By reducing the intake of foods that create an acidic environment, the diet supports the body's natural defenses. Alkaline foods are typically high in vitamins and minerals that boost immune function, such as vitamin C, vitamin E, and zinc. A robust immune system is better equipped to fend off infections and illnesses, ensuring better health and resilience.

Bone health is another critical area positively affected by the alkaline diet. Contrary to the conventional belief that dairy products are the best source of calcium, the alkaline diet highlights plant-based sources such as leafy greens, almonds, and sesame seeds. These foods not only provide adequate calcium but also help maintain an optimal pH balance, which is essential for preserving bone density. Acidic diets can leach calcium from the bones to neutralize excess acid, leading to weakened bones over time. The alkaline diet prevents this by promoting a natural pH balance that supports bone strength and health. Adopting an alkaline diet can also lead to better sleep patterns. Many individuals find that the reduction in inflammatory foods and the increase in nutrient-dense, alkaline foods help improve the quality of their sleep. Better sleep quality contributes to overall health, enhancing everything from cognitive function to physical recovery and emotional stability. The overarching benefit of the alkaline diet is its holistic approach to health. By focusing on the consumption of natural, whole foods and avoiding those that create acid, the diet supports the body in achieving and maintaining a state of balance and optimal functioning. This holistic approach does not merely target specific symptoms or conditions but rather promotes an overall sense of well-being and vitality.

In essence, the alkaline diet is not just about what you eat but how those choices impact your entire body. It is a comprehensive lifestyle change that encourages mindful eating and an appreciation for the natural benefits of food. By fostering a balanced internal environment, the alkaline diet helps you feel more vibrant, energized, and resilient, ready to face the challenges of everyday life with a renewed sense of health and well-being.

Detailed Diet Plans

Daily and Weekly Plans

Embarking on an alkaline diet requires a thoughtful approach to meal planning. By focusing on foods that promote an optimal pH balance in the body, you can achieve significant health benefits. Crafting daily and weekly meal plans ensures that you maintain variety, enjoy delicious meals, and stay committed to the dietary principles set forth by Dr. Sebi. Let's delve into the structure of these plans, considering the unique aspects that make the alkaline diet both effective and enjoyable.

When you begin planning your daily meals, it's crucial to start with breakfast, as it sets the tone for your day. An ideal alkaline breakfast is both nutrient-dense and satisfying. Consider starting your day with a smoothie made from leafy greens like kale or spinach, combined with alkaline fruits such as apples, pears, and berries. Adding a tablespoon of chia seeds or flaxseeds not only boosts the nutrient content but also provides essential omega-3 fatty acids. If you prefer a more substantial breakfast, a quinoa porridge, topped with fresh fruits and a sprinkle of nuts, offers a warm, comforting start to your day while adhering to alkaline principles.

As you transition to lunch, the goal is to keep the meal light yet packed with nutrients to sustain your energy levels throughout the afternoon. A large salad with a base of mixed greens, such as arugula, watercress, and romaine lettuce, serves as an excellent foundation. Top it with colorful vegetables like bell peppers, cucumbers, and cherry tomatoes. For added protein, incorporate avocado slices, chickpeas, or a handful of almonds. Dress your salad with a simple lemon-tahini dressing, which not only enhances the flavor but also keeps the meal alkaline-friendly. Alternatively, a vegetable stir-fry featuring zucchini, bell peppers, onions, and snap peas, served over a bed of quinoa or wild rice, can provide a warm and satisfying lunch option.

Dinner on the alkaline diet should be nourishing yet not too heavy, allowing for easy digestion before bedtime. Consider preparing a vegetable soup made with a rich broth of blended tomatoes, carrots, and celery, seasoned with herbs like basil, oregano, and thyme. Add chunks of vegetables such as zucchini, squash, and kale for added texture and nutrition. Pair this with a side of roasted sweet potatoes and a serving of steamed broccoli to create a well-rounded evening meal. Another option is a baked portobello mushroom stuffed with a mixture of quinoa, spinach, and pine nuts, served alongside a mixed vegetable medley.

Transitioning to a weekly meal plan, it's beneficial to structure your days to ensure variety and balance. On Mondays, you might start with a green smoothie for breakfast, a quinoa and vegetable salad for lunch, and a hearty vegetable soup for dinner. Tuesdays could feature a chia seed pudding with berries for breakfast, a wrap filled with hummus, avocado, and mixed greens for lunch, and a zucchini noodle pasta with a tomato-basil sauce for dinner.

Wednesdays can be a day to enjoy a fresh fruit platter for breakfast, a tabbouleh salad with parsley, tomatoes, and quinoa for lunch, and a baked sweet potato topped with sautéed spinach and mushrooms for dinner. Thursdays might include an almond milk smoothie bowl with fruits and nuts for breakfast, a lentil and vegetable stew for lunch, and a stuffed bell pepper with a side of steamed asparagus for dinner.

Fridays can kick off with a hearty oatmeal made with almond milk and topped with sliced bananas and chia seeds. For lunch, a mixed bean salad with chickpeas, black beans, and kidney beans, dressed with a lemon vinaigrette, provides a protein-packed option. Dinner could be a cauliflower and broccoli bake, seasoned with garlic and herbs, served with a side of quinoa.

As the weekend approaches, Saturdays might start with a fresh vegetable juice, followed by a mid-morning snack of apple slices with almond butter. Lunch could be a marinated tofu stir-fry with mixed vegetables, and dinner a baked acorn squash stuffed with a wild rice and vegetable mixture. Sundays can be a day for a more leisurely breakfast, perhaps an avocado toast on spelt bread with a sprinkle of hemp seeds, a hearty vegetable and lentil soup for lunch, and a final dinner of the week featuring a roasted vegetable platter with a side of quinoa.

To maintain variety and prevent meal fatigue, it's important to rotate your vegetables, grains, and protein sources. This not only ensures a broad spectrum of nutrients but also keeps your meals exciting and flavorful. For instance, if you've had quinoa several times during the week, try amaranth or millet as a grain alternative. Similarly, swap out chickpeas for lentils or black beans in your salads and stews to keep your palate engaged.

Meal prepping can be a valuable strategy in adhering to your alkaline diet. Setting aside time each week to chop vegetables, cook grains, and prepare dressings can streamline your daily meal preparation, making it easier to stick to your dietary goals. Investing in quality storage containers can help keep your prepped ingredients fresh and ready to use.

Hydration plays a vital role in the alkaline diet. Drinking plenty of water, herbal teas, and fresh vegetable juices throughout the day supports the body's natural detoxification processes and helps maintain the desired pH balance. Adding a squeeze of lemon to your water not only enhances flavor but also promotes alkalinity.

Lastly, while meal planning is essential, it's also important to listen to your body. Cravings and hunger cues can provide insight into what your body needs at any given time. The alkaline diet is flexible enough to accommodate these needs, allowing you to adjust your meal plan as necessary. If you find yourself craving something sweet, a fresh fruit salad or a smoothie can satisfy that desire in a healthy, alkaline-friendly way.

Creating a daily and weekly meal plan for the alkaline diet involves thoughtful consideration of food choices and preparation methods. By emphasizing fresh, whole foods and rotating ingredients, you can enjoy a varied and nutritious diet that supports optimal health. Whether through vibrant salads, hearty soups, or creative grain dishes, the alkaline diet offers a delicious and sustainable way to nourish your body and maintain a balanced pH. Through careful planning and mindful eating, you can fully embrace the benefits of this dietary approach, leading to enhanced well-being and vitality.

Sample Menus for Breakfast, Lunch, and Dinner

Creating a variety of delicious, balanced meals is crucial for maintaining an alkaline diet. These sample menus for breakfast, lunch, and dinner not only follow the principles of the alkaline diet but also ensure that every meal is enjoyable and satisfying. Each meal is crafted to provide essential nutrients while maintaining the body's optimal pH balance.

Breakfast is often considered the most important meal of the day, and on the alkaline diet, it sets the stage for sustained energy and focus. One delightful option is an acai berry smoothie bowl. Blend frozen acai berries with a banana, a handful of spinach, and some almond milk until smooth. Pour the mixture into a bowl and top it with fresh berries, sliced kiwi, chia seeds, and a sprinkle of granola. This vibrant and nutrient-dense breakfast not only boosts energy levels but also provides antioxidants and fiber to start the day on a healthy note.

For those who prefer a savory breakfast, a veggie scramble with tofu can be a fantastic choice. Crumble firm tofu into a skillet with a little olive oil, then add chopped bell peppers, onions, spinach, and tomatoes. Season with turmeric, cumin, and a pinch of sea salt. Serve with a side of avocado slices and a piece of toasted spelt bread. This protein-rich meal keeps you full and satisfied, offering a hearty start without compromising your alkaline diet.

As the day progresses, lunch should be both light and nourishing, keeping you energized without causing that mid-afternoon slump. A quinoa and roasted vegetable salad fits the bill perfectly. Prepare by roasting a mix of vegetables such as zucchini, bell peppers, carrots, and cherry tomatoes with a drizzle of olive oil and a sprinkle of sea salt. Once roasted, combine them with cooked quinoa and toss with a lemon-tahini dressing. Add a handful of fresh arugula and a sprinkle of toasted sunflower seeds for added crunch. This meal is not only visually appealing but also packed with vitamins, minerals, and plant-based protein.

Another excellent lunch option is a Mediterranean chickpea salad. Combine chickpeas with diced cucumbers, cherry tomatoes, red onions, and Kalamata olives. Toss with fresh parsley, a squeeze of lemon juice, a splash of olive oil, and a dash of sea salt and black pepper. Serve on a bed of mixed greens with a side of whole grain pita. This refreshing and flavorful salad is rich in fiber and healthy fats, making it a satisfying midday meal.

Dinner should be a time to relax and enjoy a comforting, yet healthful, meal. A stuffed bell pepper dish can be both satisfying and aligned with the alkaline diet. Start by cutting the tops off of red or yellow bell peppers and removing the seeds. In a skillet, sauté onions, garlic, and chopped mushrooms until tender. Add cooked quinoa, black beans, corn, and diced tomatoes, seasoning with cumin, paprika, and a pinch of sea salt. Stuff the peppers with this mixture and bake in the oven until the peppers are tender. Serve with a side of steamed broccoli or a simple mixed green salad. This dish is rich in flavor and texture, making it a perfect evening meal.

For a simpler dinner option, consider a hearty vegetable soup. Begin by sautéing onions, garlic, and celery in a large pot with a little olive oil. Add diced carrots, sweet potatoes, zucchini, and kale. Pour in vegetable broth and bring to a simmer. Season with bay leaves, thyme, and a pinch of sea salt. Allow the soup to cook until all the vegetables are tender. Serve with a slice of whole grain bread or a side of quinoa for a complete meal. This comforting soup is easy to prepare and perfect for a relaxing dinner after a long day.

Incorporating a variety of dishes throughout the week ensures that meals remain exciting and nutritionally balanced. For breakfast, consider alternating between smoothie bowls, veggie scrambles, and even overnight oats. To make overnight oats, combine rolled oats with almond milk, chia seeds, and a touch of maple syrup in a jar. Let it sit in the refrigerator overnight, and in the morning, top with fresh berries and a handful of nuts. This quick and convenient breakfast can be prepared the night before, making it ideal for busy mornings.

Lunches can vary between hearty salads, wraps, and soups. A collard green wrap is a fun and nutritious option. Use large collard green leaves as the wrap and fill with hummus, shredded carrots, cucumber slices, avocado, and a sprinkle of sunflower seeds. Roll up and enjoy a crunchy, flavorful lunch that's easy to pack for work or school.

Dinners can feature an array of comforting dishes that adhere to the alkaline principles. A vegetable stir-fry with brown rice is a versatile option. In a hot skillet, stir-fry broccoli, snap peas, bell peppers, and mushrooms in a little sesame oil. Add a splash of tamari or coconut aminos for flavor. Serve over a bed of brown rice or quinoa for a filling and nutritious meal.

For a more elaborate dinner, try a baked eggplant dish. Slice eggplants lengthwise and bake until tender. Top with a homemade tomato sauce made from sautéing garlic, onions, tomatoes, and fresh basil. Sprinkle with nutritional yeast for a cheesy flavor and bake until bubbly. Serve with a side of sautéed spinach and a slice of whole grain bread. This meal is not only delicious but also showcases the versatility of plant-based ingredients in creating satisfying dishes.

Throughout the week, it's important to stay hydrated and incorporate snacks that align with the alkaline diet. Fresh fruits, raw vegetables with hummus, and a handful of nuts or seeds make excellent snacks that keep you energized between meals. Herbal teas and infused waters with lemon or cucumber slices can also help maintain hydration and support overall health.

Adopting these sample menus for breakfast, lunch, and dinner provides a clear path to enjoying a balanced, alkaline diet. Each meal is designed to be flavorful, nutrient-dense, and satisfying, ensuring that you can stick to the diet with ease. By planning your meals in advance and incorporating a variety of ingredients, you can enjoy the benefits of the alkaline diet while delighting in a range of delicious dishes. Whether it's a vibrant smoothie bowl, a hearty quinoa salad, or a comforting vegetable soup, each meal contributes to your overall well-being and pH balance, making the alkaline diet both practical and enjoyable.

Alkaline Recipes

Smoothies and Juices

Incorporating smoothies and juices into your daily routine is a delightful way to embrace the alkaline diet. These beverages are not only refreshing but also packed with nutrients that promote optimal health and maintain the body's pH balance. Here are three invigorating recipes that are both easy to prepare and incredibly nourishing.

Green Power Smoothie

- Preparation time: 10 minutes
- Ingredients:
    - 1 cup of spinach
    - 1 cup of kale, stems removed
    - 1 green apple, cored and chopped
    - 1 banana
    - 1 tablespoon of chia seeds
    - 1 tablespoon of almond butter
    - 1 cup of almond milk
    - Juice of 1 lemon
- Portions: 2 servings

Procedure:

1. Begin by washing the spinach and kale thoroughly to remove any dirt or pesticides.

2. Core and chop the green apple into manageable pieces. Peel the banana and break it into chunks.

3. In a high-speed blender, combine the spinach, kale, apple, banana, chia seeds, almond butter, almond milk, and lemon juice.

4. Blend until smooth and creamy, ensuring that no large pieces of greens remain.

5. Pour into glasses and enjoy immediately for the freshest taste and maximum nutritional benefit.

The Green Power Smoothie is a perfect morning pick-me-up, providing a substantial dose of vitamins, minerals, and healthy fats. The combination of spinach and kale offers a robust base of iron and calcium, while the apple add a touch of natural.

Berry Bliss Juice

- Preparation time: 10 minutes
- Ingredients:
    - 1 cup of strawberries, hulled
    - 1 cup of blueberries
    - 1 cup of raspberries
    - 1 cup of coconut water
    - 1 tablespoon of flaxseeds
    - 1 tablespoon of agave syrup (optional)
- Portions: 2 servings

Procedure:

1. Wash the berries thoroughly under cold water.

2. Hull the strawberries and ensure all berries are free from stems and leaves.

3. In a blender, combine the strawberries, blueberries, raspberries, coconut water, flaxseeds, and agave syrup if you prefer a sweeter juice.

4. Blend until the mixture is smooth and well combined.

5. Strain the juice through a fine mesh sieve or cheesecloth to remove the pulp, if desired.

6. Pour the juice into glasses, add a few ice cubes if preferred, and enjoy immediately.

Berry Bliss Juice is an antioxidant powerhouse, perfect for a mid-afternoon refreshment or a post-workout boost. Berries are rich in vitamins C and E, which are crucial for skin health and immune function. Coconut water adds a hydrating element, while flaxseeds offer additional fiber and omega-3 fatty acids, promoting heart and brain health. This juice is light, refreshing, and packed with essential nutrients.

Citrus Sunshine Smoothie

- Preparation time: 10 minutes
- Ingredients:
    - 2 oranges, peeled and segmented
    - 1 grapefruit, peeled and segmented
    - 1 carrot, peeled and chopped
    - 1-inch piece of ginger, peeled
    - 1 tablespoon of hemp seeds
    - 1 cup of coconut milk
    - Juice of 1 lime
- Portions: 2 servings
- Procedure:

1. Peel and segment the oranges and grapefruit, removing any seeds.

2. Peel and chop the carrot into small pieces.

3. Peel the ginger and chop it into smaller pieces to facilitate blending.

4. In a blender, combine the oranges, grapefruit, carrot, ginger, hemp seeds, coconut milk, and lime juice.

5. Blend on high speed until the mixture is smooth and frothy.

6. Pour the smoothie into glasses and serve immediately, savoring the bright and zesty flavors.

Tropical Paradise Smoothie

- Preparation time: 10 minutes
- Ingredients:
    - 1 cup of fresh pineapple chunks
    - 1 mango, peeled and diced
    - 1 banana
    - 1 cup of coconut water
    - 1 tablespoon of flaxseeds
    - 1 cup of spinach
    - Juice of 1 lime
- Portions: 2 servings

Procedure:

1. Peel and dice the mango, and chop the pineapple into chunks.

2. Peel the banana and break it into pieces.

3. Wash the spinach thoroughly.

4. Combine the pineapple, mango, banana, coconut water, flaxseeds, spinach, and lime juice in a blender.

5. Blend until smooth and creamy.

6. Pour into glasses and enjoy immediately for a refreshing tropical treat.

The Tropical Paradise Smoothie is like a vacation in a glass. Pineapple and mango add natural sweetness and a burst of tropical flavor, while spinach provides a hidden boost of nutrients. Flaxseeds add omega-3 fatty acids, and coconut water hydrates and refreshes.

Beetroot Blast Juice

- Preparation time: 10 minutes

- Ingredients:

    - 2 medium beets, peeled and chopped

    - 2 carrots, peeled and chopped

    - 1 apple, cored and chopped

    - 1-inch piece of ginger, peeled

    - 1 lemon, peeled

    - 1 cup of water

- Portions: 2 servings

- Procedure:

1. Peel and chop the beets, carrots, and apple.

2. Peel the ginger and chop it into smaller pieces.

3. Peel the lemon, removing as much white pith as possible.

4. Combine the beets, carrots, apple, ginger, lemon, and water in a blender.

5. Blend until smooth.

6. Strain the mixture through a fine mesh sieve or cheesecloth to remove the pulp, if desired.

7. Pour the juice into glasses and enjoy immediately.

Beetroot Blast Juice is a vibrant and nutrient-packed drink. Beets are rich in antioxidants and nitrates, which can help improve blood flow and lower blood pressure. Carrots add sweetness and beta-carotene, while ginger and lemon provide a zesty kick.

Creamy Avocado Smoothie

- Preparation time: 10 minutes
- Ingredients:
    - 1 ripe avocado
    - 1 banana
    - 1 cup of almond milk
    - 1 tablespoon of hemp seeds
    - 1 teaspoon of vanilla extract
    - 1 tablespoon of agave syrup (optional)
- Portions: 2 servings
- Procedure:

1. Cut the avocado in half, remove the pit, and scoop the flesh into the blender.

2. Peel the banana and break it into chunks.

3. Combine the avocado, banana, almond milk, hemp seeds, vanilla extract, and agave syrup in a blender.

4. Blend until smooth and creamy.

5. Pour into glasses and enjoy immediately.

The Creamy Avocado Smoothie is rich, smooth, and incredibly satisfying. Avocado provides healthy fats and a creamy texture, while banana adds natural sweetness. Hemp seeds contribute protein and essential fatty acids, making this smoothie both delicious and nutritious.

Cucumber Mint Cooler

- Preparation time: 10 minutes

- Ingredients:

  - 1 large cucumber, peeled and chopped

  - 1 handful of fresh mint leaves

  - 1 green apple, cored and chopped

  - 1 lemon, peeled

  - 1 cup of coconut water

- Portions: 2 servings

- Procedure:

1. Peel and chop the cucumber.

2. Wash the mint leaves thoroughly.

3. Core and chop the green apple.

4. Peel the lemon, removing as much white pith as possible.

5. Combine the cucumber, mint leaves, green apple, lemon, and coconut water in a blender.

6. Blend until smooth.

7. Strain the mixture through a fine mesh sieve or cheesecloth to remove the pulp, if desired.

8. Pour the juice into glasses and enjoy immediately.

The Cucumber Mint Cooler is a refreshing and hydrating drink, perfect for hot days. Cucumber and mint provide a cooling effect, while green apple and lemon add a touch of sweetness and tanginess. Coconut water hydrates and balances electrolytes.

Pineapple Spinach Smoothie

- Preparation time: 10 minutes
- Ingredients:
    - 1 cup of fresh pineapple chunks
    - 1 cup of spinach
    - 1 banana
    - 1 cup of coconut milk
    - 1 tablespoon of chia seeds
    - Juice of 1 lemon
- Portions: 2 servings
- Procedure:

1. Chop the pineapple into chunks.

2. Wash the spinach thoroughly.

3. Peel the banana and break it into pieces.

4. Combine the pineapple, spinach, banana, coconut milk, chia seeds, and lemon juice in a blender.

5. Blend until smooth and creamy.

6. Pour into glasses and enjoy immediately.

The Pineapple Spinach Smoothie is a nutrient-dense drink with a perfect balance of sweetness and greens. Pineapple adds a tropical flair, while spinach boosts the nutritional content without overpowering the flavor. Chia seeds add texture and essential nutrients.

Apple Carrot Ginger Juice

- Preparation time: 10 minutes
- Ingredients:
  - 2 apples, cored and chopped
  - 3 carrots, peeled and chopped
  - 1-inch piece of ginger, peeled
  - 1 lemon, peeled
  - 1 cup of water
- Portions: 2 servings
- Procedure:

1. Core and chop the apples.

2. Peel and chop the carrots.

3. Peel the ginger and chop it into smaller pieces.

4. Peel the lemon, removing as much white pith as possible.

5. Combine the apples, carrots, ginger, lemon, and water in a blender.

6. Blend until smooth.

7. Strain the mixture through a fine mesh sieve or cheesecloth to remove the pulp, if desired.

8. Pour the juice into glasses and enjoy immediately.

The Apple Carrot Ginger Juice is a classic combination that is both refreshing and invigorating. Apples and carrots provide natural sweetness and a host of vitamins, while ginger adds a spicy kick that aids digestion and boosts immunity.

Blueberry Kale Smoothie

- Preparation time: 10 minutes
- Ingredients:
  - 1 cup of blueberries
  - 1 cup of kale, stems removed
  - 1 banana
  - 1 cup of almond milk
  - 1 tablespoon of flaxseeds
  - 1 tablespoon of agave syrup (optional)
- Portions: 2 servings
- Procedure:

1. Wash the blueberries and kale thoroughly.

2. Remove the stems from the kale.

3. Peel the banana and break it into chunks.

4. Combine the blueberries, kale, banana, almond milk, flaxseeds, and agave syrup in a blender.

5. Blend until smooth and creamy.

6. Pour into glasses and enjoy immediately.

The Blueberry Kale Smoothie is a powerhouse of antioxidants and nutrients. Blueberries add sweetness and a beautiful color, while kale provides a wealth of vitamins and minerals. Flaxseeds add omega-3 fatty acids, enhancing the nutritional profile of this delicious smoothie.

Main meals

Crafting delicious and nutritious main meals is a cornerstone of the alkaline diet. These recipes not only adhere to alkaline principles but also deliver a variety of flavors and textures that will keep your palate excited and satisfied. Here are ten recipes that make perfect main meals, each designed to promote health and balance.

Recipe 1: Quinoa Stuffed Bell Peppers

- Preparation time: 45 minutes
- Ingredients:

  - 4 bell peppers, tops cut off and seeds removed
  - 1 cup quinoa, rinsed
  - 2 cups vegetable broth
  - 1 small onion, finely chopped
  - 1 zucchini, diced
  - 1 cup cherry tomatoes, halved
  - 1 cup black beans, drained and rinsed
  - 1 tablespoon olive oil
  - 1 teaspoon cumin
  - 1 teaspoon smoked paprika
  - Sea salt and black pepper to taste

- Portions: 4 servings
- Procedure:

1. Preheat your oven to 375°F (190°C). In a pot, bring vegetable broth to a boil. Add quinoa, reduce heat, cover, and simmer for 15 minutes until the quinoa is cooked.

2. In a skillet, heat olive oil over medium heat. Sauté onion until translucent, then add zucchini and cook for 5 minutes.

3. Stir in cherry tomatoes, black beans, cumin, smoked paprika, salt, and pepper. Cook for another 3 minutes. Combine the cooked quinoa with the vegetable mixture.

4. Stuff each bell pepper with the quinoa mixture and place them in a baking dish.

5. Cover with foil and bake for 30 minutes. Remove foil for the last 10 minutes to lightly brown the tops.

6. Serve hot and enjoy a nutritious, colorful meal.

Recipe 2: Zucchini Noodles with Avocado Pesto

- Preparation time: 20 minutes
- Ingredients:
  - 4 large zucchinis
  - 2 ripe avocados
  - 1 cup fresh basil leaves
  - 2 cloves garlic
  - 1/4 cup pine nuts
  - 1/4 cup olive oil
  - Juice of 1 lemon
  - Sea salt and black pepper to taste
- Portions: 4 servings
- Procedure:

1. Spiralize the zucchinis to create noodles and set aside.

2. In a food processor, combine avocados, basil, garlic, pine nuts, olive oil, lemon juice, salt, and pepper. Blend until smooth.

3. Toss the zucchini noodles with the avocado pesto until well coated.

4. Serve immediately, garnished with extra pine nuts and basil leaves.

Recipe 3: Lentil and Vegetable Stew

- Preparation time: 1 hour
- Ingredients:
    - 1 cup green lentils, rinsed
    - 1 onion, chopped
    - 2 carrots, diced
    - 2 celery stalks, chopped
    - 1 zucchini, chopped
    - 1 can diced tomatoes
    - 4 cups vegetable broth
    - 2 cloves garlic, minced
    - 1 teaspoon thyme
    - 1 teaspoon rosemary
    - Sea salt and black pepper to taste
- Portions: 6 servings
- Procedure:

1. In a large pot, sauté onion, carrots, and celery in olive oil until softened.
2. Add garlic, thyme, and rosemary, and cook for another minute.
3. Stir in lentils, diced tomatoes, and vegetable broth. Bring to a boil.
4. Reduce heat and simmer for 35-40 minutes until lentils are tender.
5. Add zucchini and cook for an additional 10 minutes.
6. Season with salt and pepper, and serve hot.

Recipe 4: Chickpea and Spinach Curry

- Preparation time: 30 minutes
- Ingredients:
    - 1 can chickpeas, drained and rinsed
    - 1 onion, finely chopped
    - 2 cloves garlic, minced
    - 1 inch piece of ginger, grated
    - 1 can coconut milk
    - 1 cup vegetable broth
    - 3 cups fresh spinach, chopped
    - 2 tablespoons curry powder
    - 1 teaspoon turmeric
    - 1 teaspoon cumin
    - Sea salt and black pepper to taste
- Portions: 4 servings
- Procedure:

1. In a large pan, sauté onion, garlic, and ginger in olive oil until fragrant.
2. Add curry powder, turmeric, and cumin, and cook for another minute.
3. Stir in chickpeas, coconut milk, and vegetable broth. Bring to a simmer.
4. Add spinach and cook until wilted, about 5 minutes.
5. Season with salt and pepper, and serve over brown rice or quinoa.

Recipe 5: Sweet Potato and Black Bean Tacos

- Preparation time: 30 minutes

- Ingredients:

    - 2 large sweet potatoes, peeled and diced

    - 1 can black beans, drained and rinsed

    - 1 teaspoon cumin

    - 1 teaspoon smoked paprika

    - 8 small corn tortillas

    - 1 avocado, sliced

    - 1 cup shredded red cabbage

    - 1 lime, cut into wedges

    - Sea salt and black pepper to taste

- Portions: 4 servings

- Procedure:

1.   Preheat oven to 400°F (200°C).

2.   Toss sweet potatoes with olive oil, cumin, smoked paprika, salt, and pepper. Spread on a baking sheet and roast for 20 minutes until tender.

3.   Warm the tortillas in a dry skillet or oven.

4.   Fill each tortilla with roasted sweet potatoes, black beans, avocado slices, and shredded cabbage.

5.   Serve with lime wedges for squeezing over the tacos.

Recipe 6: Cauliflower Fried Rice

- Preparation time: 25 minutes
- Ingredients:
    - 1 head of cauliflower, riced
    - 1 cup frozen peas and carrots
    - 1 bell pepper, diced
    - 1 small onion, chopped
    - 2 cloves garlic, minced
    - 2 tablespoons soy sauce or tamari
    - 2 eggs, lightly beaten
    - 2 tablespoons sesame oil
    - 2 green onions, sliced
- Portions: 4 servings
- Procedure:

1. Heat sesame oil in a large skillet over medium heat. Sauté onion and garlic until fragrant.

2. Add bell pepper and cook for 3 minutes.

3. Stir in cauliflower rice and cook for another 5 minutes.

4. Push vegetables to the side and pour eggs into the skillet. Scramble until cooked through, then mix with the vegetables.

5. Add frozen peas and carrots, soy sauce, and cook until heated through.

6. Garnish with sliced green onions and serve.

Recipe 7: Eggplant and Tomato Bake

- Preparation time: 45 minutes
- Ingredients:
    - 2 large eggplants, sliced
    - 4 large tomatoes, sliced
    - 1 onion, thinly sliced
    - 4 cloves garlic, minced
    - 1/4 cup olive oil
    - 1 teaspoon oregano
    - 1 teaspoon thyme
    - Sea salt and black pepper to taste
    - Fresh basil leaves for garnish
- Portions: 4 servings
- Procedure:

1. Preheat oven to 375°F (190°C).

2. Arrange eggplant and tomato slices in a baking dish, alternating between the two.

3. Scatter sliced onions and minced garlic over the top.

4. Drizzle with olive oil and sprinkle with oregano, thyme, salt, and pepper.

5. Cover with foil and bake for 30 minutes. Remove foil and bake for another 10 minutes until vegetables are tender.

6. Garnish with fresh basil leaves before serving.

Recipe 8: Spaghetti Squash with Tomato Basil Sauce

- Preparation time: 40 minutes

- Ingredients:

    - 1 large spaghetti squash

    - 4 cups cherry tomatoes, halved

    - 1 small onion, chopped

    - 3 cloves garlic, minced

    - 1/4 cup olive oil

    - 1/2 cup fresh basil, chopped

    - Sea salt and black pepper to taste

- Portions: 4 servings

- Procedure:

1.   Preheat oven to 400°F (200°C).

2.   Cut the spaghetti squash in half and remove seeds. Drizzle with olive oil and season with salt and pepper.

3.   Place squash cut-side down on a baking sheet and roast for 30 minutes until tender.

4.   In a skillet, heat olive oil and sauté onion and garlic until fragrant.

5.   Add cherry tomatoes and cook until they begin to break down.

6.   Stir in fresh basil, salt, and pepper.

7.   Scrape out the spaghetti squash strands and toss with the tomato basil sauce.

8.   Serve immediately, garnished with additional basil if desired.

Recipe 9: Vegetable Stir-Fry with Tempeh

- Preparation time: 30 minutes

- Ingredients:
    - 1 block tempeh, cubed
    - 1 red bell pepper, sliced
    - 1 yellow bell pepper, sliced
    - 1 cup broccoli florets
    - 1 carrot, julienned
    - 1 zucchini, sliced
    - 2 cloves garlic, minced
    - 1/4 cup soy sauce or tamari
    - 2 tablespoons sesame oil
    - 1 tablespoon grated ginger
    - 1 teaspoon maple syrup
    - 2 green onions, sliced
    - Sesame seeds for garnish

- Portions: 4 servings

- Procedure:

1. Heat sesame oil in a large skillet or wok over medium-high heat.

2. Add cubed tempeh and cook until golden brown on all sides.

3. Remove tempeh and set aside.

4. In the same skillet, add garlic and ginger, and cook until fragrant.

5. Add bell peppers, broccoli, carrot, and zucchini. Stir-fry for 5-7 minutes until vegetables are tender-crisp.

6. Return tempeh to the skillet and stir in soy sauce and maple syrup. Cook for another 2 minutes.

7. Garnish with sliced green onions and sesame seeds before serving.

Recipe 10: Mushroom and Spinach Quinoa

- Preparation time: 30 minutes

- Ingredients:

    - 1 cup quinoa, rinsed

    - 2 cups vegetable broth

    - 1 tablespoon olive oil

    - 1 onion, chopped

    - 2 cloves garlic, minced

    - 2 cups mushrooms, sliced

    - 3 cups fresh spinach

    - 1 teaspoon thyme

    - Sea salt and black pepper to taste

    - 1/4 cup nutritional yeast (optional)

- Portions: 4 servings

- Procedure:

1.   In a pot, bring vegetable broth to a boil. Add quinoa, reduce heat, cover, and simmer for 15 minutes until quinoa is cooked.

2.   In a skillet, heat olive oil over medium heat. Sauté onion and garlic until fragrant.

3.   Add mushrooms and cook until they release their moisture and begin to brown.

4.   Stir in fresh spinach and cook until wilted.

5.   Add cooked quinoa, thyme, salt, and pepper. Mix well.

6.   Sprinkle with nutritional yeast if desired, and serve hot.

These ten recipes showcase the versatility and deliciousness of the alkaline diet, offering a range of flavors and textures that make mealtime something to look forward to. From hearty stews and stir-fries to vibrant stuffed vegetables and creamy pasta alternatives, each dish is crafted to nourish your body and delight your taste buds. Enjoy the process of creating these meals and the benefits they bring to your health and well-being.

Snacks and Desserts

Indulging in snacks and desserts while maintaining an alkaline diet is not only possible but also delightful. By using nutrient-dense, alkaline-friendly ingredients, you can create satisfying treats that nourish your body and satisfy your cravings. Here are eight delicious recipes for snacks and desserts that align with the principles of the alkaline diet.

Recipe 1: Almond Butter Energy Balls

- Preparation time: 15 minutes

- Ingredients:

    - 1 cup rolled oats

    - 1/2 cup almond butter

    - 1/4 cup flaxseeds

    - 1/4 cup maple syrup

    - 1/4 cup shredded coconut

    - 1 teaspoon vanilla extract

    - 1/4 cup dark chocolate chips (optional)

- Portions: 12 balls

- Procedure:

1.   In a large mixing bowl, combine rolled oats, almond butter, flaxseeds, maple syrup, shredded coconut, vanilla extract, and chocolate chips if using.

2.   Mix well until all ingredients are thoroughly combined.

3.   Using your hands, roll the mixture into 1-inch balls.

4.   Place the energy balls on a baking sheet lined with parchment paper.

5.   Refrigerate for at least 30 minutes to set.

6.   Store in an airtight container in the refrigerator for up to a week.

Almond Butter Energy Balls are the perfect snack for a quick energy boost. They combine healthy fats, fiber, and a touch of sweetness, making them a great option for satisfying hunger between meals.

Recipe 2: Chia Seed Pudding

- Preparation time: 10 minutes (plus 4 hours to set)
- Ingredients:
    - 1/4 cup chia seeds
    - 1 cup almond milk
    - 1 tablespoon maple syrup
    - 1 teaspoon vanilla extract
    - Fresh berries for topping
- Portions: 2 servings
- Procedure:

1. In a bowl, whisk together chia seeds, almond milk, maple syrup, and vanilla extract.

2. Let the mixture sit for 10 minutes, then whisk again to prevent clumping.

3. Cover the bowl and refrigerate for at least 4 hours or overnight.

4. Stir the pudding before serving and top with fresh berries.

Recipe 3: Kale Chips

- Preparation time: 25 minutes
- Ingredients:
    - 1 bunch of kale
    - 2 tablespoons olive oil
    - 1 teaspoon sea salt
    - 1 teaspoon nutritional yeast (optional)
- Portions: 4 servings
- Procedure:

1. Preheat your oven to 300°F (150°C).

2. Wash and thoroughly dry the kale. Remove the stems and tear the leaves into bite-sized pieces.

3. In a large bowl, toss the kale with olive oil, sea salt, and nutritional yeast if using.

4. Spread the kale pieces in a single layer on a baking sheet.

5. Bake for 20 minutes, or until the kale is crispy, stirring halfway through.

6. Let the kale chips cool before serving.

Recipe 4: Coconut Macaroons

- Preparation time: 30 minutes

- Ingredients:

    - 2 cups shredded coconut

    - 1/4 cup almond flour

    - 1/4 cup maple syrup

    - 1 teaspoon vanilla extract

    - 1/4 teaspoon sea salt

- Portions: 12 macaroons

- Procedure:

1. Preheat your oven to 325°F (165°C).

2. In a mixing bowl, combine shredded coconut, almond flour, maple syrup, vanilla extract, and sea salt.

3. Mix until all ingredients are well incorporated.

4. Using a tablespoon, scoop out the mixture and shape it into small mounds.

5. Place the macaroons on a baking sheet lined with parchment paper.

6. Bake for 20 minutes, or until the edges are golden brown.

7. Allow the macaroons to cool completely before serving.

Coconut Macaroons are a sweet, chewy treat that's perfect for dessert. They're easy to make and packed with the delicious flavor of coconut, making them a favorite for anyone with a sweet tooth.

Recipe 5: Avocado Chocolate Mousse

- Preparation time: 10 minutes
- Ingredients:
    - 2 ripe avocados
    - 1/4 cup cocoa powder
    - 1/4 cup maple syrup
    - 1 teaspoon vanilla extract
    - A pinch of sea salt
- Portions: 4 servings
- Procedure:

1. In a food processor, combine avocados, cocoa powder, maple syrup, vanilla extract, and sea salt.

2. Blend until smooth and creamy, scraping down the sides as needed.

3. Spoon the mousse into serving bowls and refrigerate for at least 30 minutes before serving.

Avocado Chocolate Mousse is a rich, decadent dessert that's surprisingly healthy. The avocados provide a creamy texture and are rich in healthy fats, while the cocoa powder adds a deep, chocolatey flavor.

Recipe 6: Banana Ice Cream

- Preparation time: 10 minutes (plus time to freeze bananas)
- Ingredients:
    - 4 ripe bananas, sliced and frozen
    - 1 teaspoon vanilla extract
    - 1/4 cup almond milk (if needed)
- Portions: 4 servings
- Procedure:

1. Peel and slice the bananas, then freeze them for at least 4 hours or overnight.

2. In a food processor, blend the frozen banana slices and vanilla extract until smooth and creamy. Add almond milk if needed for a smoother texture.

3. Serve immediately for a soft-serve consistency or freeze for an additional hour for a firmer texture.

Recipe 7: Zucchini Fritters

- Preparation time: 30 minutes

- Ingredients:

    - 2 large zucchinis, grated

    - 1 small onion, finely chopped

    - 1/4 cup almond flour

    - 2 tablespoons nutritional yeast

    - 1 teaspoon garlic powder

    - 1/2 teaspoon sea salt

    - 1/4 teaspoon black pepper

    - 2 tablespoons olive oil

- Portions: 4 servings

- Procedure:

1.   Grate the zucchinis and squeeze out excess moisture using a clean kitchen towel.

2.   In a mixing bowl, combine grated zucchini, onion, almond flour, nutritional yeast, garlic powder, sea salt, and black pepper.

3.   Form the mixture into small patties.

4.   Heat olive oil in a skillet over medium heat.

5.   Cook the fritters for about 3-4 minutes on each side, until golden brown and crispy.

6.   Serve warm.

Zucchini Fritters are a savory snack that's both nutritious and delicious. They're crispy on the outside and tender on the inside, making them a perfect appetizer or snack.

Recipe 8: Baked Apple Chips

- Preparation time: 2 hours
- Ingredients:
    - 4 apples, thinly sliced
    - 1 teaspoon cinnamon
    - 1 tablespoon lemon juice
- Portions: 4 servings
- Procedure:

1. Preheat your oven to 200°F (95°C).

2. Thinly slice the apples using a mandoline or sharp knife.

3. In a bowl, toss the apple slices with cinnamon and lemon juice.

4. Arrange the apple slices in a single layer on a baking sheet lined with parchment paper.

5. Bake for 1.5 to 2 hours, flipping the slices halfway through, until the apples are dry and crispy.

6. Allow the apple chips to cool completely before serving.

Baked Apple Chips are a crunchy and naturally sweet snack that's perfect for munching throughout the day. They're easy to make and provide a satisfying crunch without any added sugar.

These snacks and desserts offer a delightful way to enjoy the benefits of the alkaline diet without sacrificing flavor or satisfaction. From sweet treats like Banana Ice Cream and Coconut Macaroons to savory options like Kale Chips and Zucchini Fritters, these recipes cater to a variety of tastes and cravings. Enjoy these creations and feel good about nourishing your body with each delicious bite.

Part 4: Detox Programs

Introduction to Detoxification

Importance of Intracellular Cleansing

Detoxification is more than just a buzzword; it's a crucial aspect of maintaining optimal health and wellness. The body, when given the right tools and environment, has a remarkable ability to cleanse itself of toxins. Intracellular cleansing, in particular, focuses on purifying the cells, which are the basic building blocks of our bodies. This process is essential for the elimination of waste products and toxins that accumulate from various sources, including environmental pollutants, dietary choices, and metabolic processes. Cells operate as the fundamental units of life, and their health directly impacts the overall functioning of the body. Intracellular cleansing aims to support these cells in their vital roles by ensuring they are not burdened by toxins and waste. When cells are free from harmful substances, they can perform their functions more efficiently, leading to improved energy levels, enhanced immunity, and overall better health.

The importance of intracellular cleansing cannot be overstated. It begins with understanding how toxins affect cellular health. Toxins can enter the body through various means: the air we breathe, the food we eat, and even the products we use on our skin. Once inside the body, these toxins can interfere with cellular processes, leading to oxidative stress and inflammation. Over time, this can cause cellular damage and contribute to the development of chronic diseases. To combat this, intracellular cleansing focuses on removing these harmful substances from within the cells. This process typically involves several key components: proper hydration, nutrient-rich foods, and specific cleansing practices such as fasting or herbal supplements. Each of these elements plays a vital role in supporting the body's natural detoxification processes.

Hydration is fundamental to intracellular cleansing. Water is essential for the body's detoxification pathways, helping to flush out toxins through the kidneys, liver, and skin. Staying well-hydrated ensures that these organs can perform their detoxifying functions effectively. Additionally, water aids in maintaining cellular integrity, allowing cells to function optimally.

Nutrient-rich foods are another cornerstone of intracellular cleansing. A diet abundant in fresh fruits, vegetables, and whole grains provides the body with the necessary vitamins, minerals, and antioxidants to combat oxidative stress and support cellular health. These foods are typically high in fiber, which aids in digestion and helps eliminate toxins from the digestive tract. Leafy greens, berries, nuts, and seeds are particularly beneficial for their high antioxidant content, which protects cells from damage and supports the detoxification process. Specific cleansing practices can also enhance intracellular detoxification. Fasting, for example, has been shown to promote autophagy, a process where the body breaks down and removes damaged cells and regenerates healthier ones. This natural cleansing mechanism is essential for maintaining cellular health and preventing the accumulation of cellular debris and toxins.

Herbal supplements can also play a supportive role in intracellular cleansing. Herbs like milk thistle, dandelion root, and turmeric have been traditionally used for their detoxifying properties. Milk thistle supports liver health, which is crucial for detoxification, while dandelion root aids in kidney function, helping to flush out toxins. Turmeric, with its anti-inflammatory properties, helps reduce oxidative stress and supports overall cellular health.

The benefits of regular detoxification extend beyond cellular health. When the body is free from toxins, it operates more efficiently, leading to increased energy levels and improved mental clarity. Many people report feeling more vibrant and focused after a detoxification program. This enhanced mental clarity is likely due to the removal of toxins that can impair cognitive function and contribute to brain fog. Detoxification also supports a healthy immune system. The immune system relies on a network of cells and organs to protect the body from infections and diseases. When the body is burdened with toxins, the immune system can become compromised, making it less effective at fighting off pathogens. Regular detoxification helps to maintain a healthy immune response by reducing the toxic load and supporting the function of immune cells.

Another significant benefit of detoxification is improved digestion. The digestive system plays a crucial role in eliminating waste and toxins from the body. A detoxification program that includes high-fiber foods and adequate hydration can support digestive health by promoting regular bowel movements and preventing constipation. This, in turn, helps to reduce the reabsorption of toxins from the digestive tract.

Detoxification can also aid in weight management. Toxins can interfere with the body's metabolism and contribute to weight gain. By removing these toxins, the body can reset its metabolic processes, making it easier to maintain a healthy weight. Additionally, detoxification programs often involve a diet that is low in processed foods and high in nutrient-dense, whole foods, which can support healthy weight loss.

Skin health is another area where detoxification can have a profound impact. The skin is the body's largest organ and plays a vital role in eliminating toxins through sweat. When the body is overloaded with toxins, it can lead to skin issues such as acne, eczema, and dullness. Detoxification helps to clear the skin by removing these toxins and supporting overall cellular health. Many people notice a clearer, more radiant complexion after completing a detox program. It's important to approach detoxification with a balanced perspective. While the benefits are numerous, it's essential to ensure that the detoxification methods chosen are safe and appropriate for your individual health needs. Consulting with a healthcare professional before starting any detox program can help ensure that it is tailored to your specific requirements and that it will be effective and safe.

In summary, intracellular cleansing is a vital component of overall health and wellness. By focusing on the health of individual cells, we can support the body's natural detoxification processes and promote optimal functioning. The benefits of regular detoxification are far-reaching, from increased energy levels and improved mental clarity to enhanced immune function and better digestion. Through proper hydration, nutrient-rich foods, and specific cleansing practices, we can help our bodies eliminate toxins and achieve a state of balance and vitality.

Benefits of Regular Detoxification

Detoxification is more than just a trend; it's a crucial practice for maintaining optimal health and well-being. Regular detoxification supports the body's natural ability to cleanse itself of harmful substances and can lead to profound improvements in both physical and mental health. Understanding the numerous benefits of detoxification helps us appreciate its importance in our daily lives.

One of the primary benefits of regular detoxification is enhanced energy levels. When the body is burdened with toxins, it has to work harder to maintain its normal functions, often leading to fatigue and sluggishness. Detoxification helps to remove these toxins, freeing up energy and allowing the body to operate more efficiently. People who regularly detoxify often report feeling more energetic, alert, and vibrant. This boost in energy can improve productivity and overall quality of life, making it easier to engage in physical activities and enjoy daily tasks. Improved digestion is another significant benefit of regular detoxification. The digestive system is responsible for breaking down food and absorbing nutrients, but it can become sluggish and less efficient when overloaded with toxins. A detoxification regimen that includes a diet rich in fiber, fresh fruits, and vegetables can support healthy digestion by promoting regular bowel movements and reducing bloating and discomfort. This can lead to better nutrient absorption and overall digestive health, allowing the body to get the most out of the foods we eat.

Detoxification also plays a vital role in supporting the immune system. The immune system is our body's defense against infections and diseases, and it can become compromised when exposed to high levels of toxins. Regular detoxification helps to reduce the toxic load on the body, giving the immune system a better chance to function effectively. This can result in fewer illnesses, quicker recovery times, and an overall improvement in health. By keeping the immune system in top shape, detoxification helps protect the body against a wide range of health issues.

Another area where detoxification shows significant benefits is mental clarity and emotional well-being. Toxins can affect brain function, leading to issues such as brain fog, poor concentration, and mood swings. Detoxification helps to clear out these toxins, resulting in improved cognitive function and emotional stability. Many people who undergo regular detoxification report better focus, sharper memory, and a more balanced mood. This mental clarity can enhance overall well-being and improve performance in both personal and professional life.

Skin health is greatly improved through regular detoxification. The skin is the body's largest organ and plays a crucial role in eliminating toxins. When the body is overloaded with toxins, it can lead to skin problems such as acne, eczema, and premature aging. Detoxification helps to clear the skin by removing toxins from the body and supporting cellular regeneration. This can result in a clearer, more radiant complexion and healthier skin overall. By maintaining a detoxified system, the skin can function more effectively as a barrier and detoxification organ. Weight management is another key benefit of regular detoxification. Toxins can interfere with the body's metabolism, making it more difficult to lose weight and maintain a healthy weight. Detoxification helps to reset the metabolism by removing these toxins and supporting healthy liver function, which is essential for fat metabolism. Additionally, many detoxification programs emphasize a diet that is low in processed foods and high in whole, nutrient-dense foods, which naturally supports weight loss and maintenance. By detoxifying the body, individuals can achieve and sustain a healthy weight more easily.

Detoxification also promotes better sleep. Toxins can disrupt sleep patterns and lead to issues such as insomnia and poor sleep quality. By removing these toxins, the body can achieve a more balanced state, resulting in improved sleep. Better sleep quality can have a cascading effect on overall health, leading to increased energy, better mood, and improved cognitive function. Regular detoxification helps to ensure that the body can rest and rejuvenate effectively during sleep.

The benefits of detoxification extend to cardiovascular health as well. Toxins can contribute to inflammation and oxidative stress, which are risk factors for heart disease. Regular detoxification helps to reduce inflammation and oxidative stress, supporting heart health. A diet that supports detoxification is typically rich in antioxidants, which protect the heart and blood vessels from damage. This can result in lower blood pressure, improved cholesterol levels, and a reduced risk of cardiovascular diseases.

Detoxification can also enhance liver function. The liver is the body's primary detoxification organ, responsible for filtering toxins from the blood and processing them for elimination. Regular detoxification supports liver health by reducing the burden of toxins that the liver has to process. This can improve the liver's efficiency and overall function, helping the body to detoxify more effectively. A healthy liver is crucial for maintaining overall health, as it plays a central role in many metabolic processes.

Moreover, detoxification supports kidney health. The kidneys filter waste products from the blood and excrete them in urine. Toxins can impair kidney function, leading to issues such as kidney stones and chronic kidney disease. Regular detoxification helps to reduce the toxic load on the kidneys, supporting their function and preventing damage. This can result in better kidney health and overall urinary tract function. Regular detoxification also contributes to hormonal balance. Toxins can disrupt the endocrine system, leading to hormonal imbalances that can affect everything from mood to metabolism to reproductive health. Detoxification helps to remove these endocrine-disrupting toxins, supporting hormonal balance and overall endocrine health. This can result in improved mood, better metabolic function, and enhanced reproductive health. In addition to these physical benefits, detoxification can also have a positive impact on mental and emotional health. The process of detoxification often involves practices such as mindfulness, meditation, and stress reduction, which can contribute to overall well-being. By focusing on both physical and mental health, detoxification can lead to a more balanced, harmonious state of being.

Overall, the benefits of regular detoxification are extensive and multifaceted. From increased energy levels and improved digestion to enhanced immune function and better mental clarity, detoxification supports every aspect of health. By incorporating regular detoxification practices into our lives, we can support our bodies in eliminating toxins, promoting optimal health, and achieving a state of balance and vitality.

Detox Programs

Fasting Guide: Water Fasting, Juice Fasting, and Fruit Fasting

Fasting is a powerful method of detoxification that has been practiced for centuries across various cultures and traditions. It involves abstaining from food for a specific period, allowing the body to rest, repair, and rejuvenate. There are several types of fasting, each with its unique benefits and challenges. Understanding the nuances of water fasting, juice fasting, and fruit fasting can help you choose the method that best suits your needs and lifestyle.

Water fasting is one of the most rigorous forms of fasting. It involves consuming only water for a set period, typically ranging from 24 hours to several days. This type of fasting gives the digestive system a complete rest, allowing the body to focus its energy on detoxification and healing. During a water fast, the body enters a state of ketosis, where it starts to burn fat for fuel, leading to the production of ketones. This metabolic shift not only aids in weight loss but also has potential benefits for brain health and cognitive function.

Water fasting can be challenging, especially for those new to fasting. It requires a strong commitment and mental preparation. It's essential to start with a shorter duration, such as a 24-hour fast, before attempting longer periods. During the fast, staying hydrated is crucial, as water helps flush out toxins from the body. Listening to your body is vital; if you experience severe discomfort or dizziness, it's essential to break the fast safely by consuming light, easily digestible foods like fruits or broths.

Juice fasting, also known as juice cleansing, is a more approachable form of fasting that involves consuming only fresh vegetable and fruit juices. This method provides the body with essential vitamins, minerals, and antioxidants while still giving the digestive system a rest. Juice fasting can last from a single day to a week or more, depending on your goals and experience. The juices should be freshly made from organic produce to maximize their nutritional benefits and avoid any harmful pesticides.

One of the significant advantages of juice fasting is that it allows for a higher intake of nutrients compared to water fasting. The juices supply the body with the necessary energy to function throughout the day while still promoting detoxification. Common ingredients for juice fasting include leafy greens, carrots, beets, apples, and citrus fruits. Adding herbs like ginger and turmeric can enhance the detoxifying effects and add flavor. It's important to consume a variety of juices to ensure a broad spectrum of nutrients and prevent monotony.

Fruit fasting is another gentle yet effective method of detoxification. This type of fasting involves consuming only fresh fruits and sometimes incorporating smoothies made from whole fruits. Fruits are naturally high in water content, fiber, and essential nutrients, making them an excellent choice for cleansing the body. Fruit fasting can be done for short durations, such as a single day, or extended to several days, depending on individual tolerance and goals.

Fruit fasting offers several benefits, including improved digestion, increased energy levels, and enhanced hydration. The natural sugars in fruits provide a steady source of energy, preventing the fatigue that sometimes accompanies fasting. Additionally, the fiber content aids in bowel regularity and supports the elimination of toxins. Popular fruits for fasting include berries, melons, apples, oranges, and grapes. It's crucial to choose organic fruits whenever possible to avoid pesticide exposure and maximize the detoxifying effects.

Embarking on a fasting journey requires careful planning and preparation. Regardless of the type of fasting chosen, it's essential to ease into the fast gradually. Reducing the intake of caffeine, processed foods, and sugar in the days leading up to the fast can help minimize withdrawal symptoms and make the transition smoother. Staying hydrated and consuming light, whole foods before starting the fast prepares the body for the cleansing process.

During the fasting period, listening to your body and paying attention to its signals is crucial. Mild hunger pangs, fatigue, and headaches are common, especially during the initial stages, as the body adjusts to the absence of solid food. However, if you experience severe discomfort, dizziness, or any other concerning symptoms, it's important to break the fast safely and consult with a healthcare professional if necessary.

Breaking the fast is as important as the fasting period itself. The digestive system needs time to readjust to solid foods, so it's essential to start with light, easily digestible meals. Fresh fruits, vegetable broths, and smoothies are excellent options for breaking a fast. Gradually reintroducing more complex foods over the next few days helps the digestive system adapt and prevents discomfort.

Each type of fasting offers unique benefits and can be tailored to individual needs and goals. Water fasting is ideal for those seeking deep cellular detoxification and a complete digestive reset. Juice fasting provides a nutrient-rich alternative that supports detoxification while supplying essential vitamins and minerals. Fruit fasting offers a gentler approach, with the added benefits of hydration and fiber.

Fasting can be a powerful tool for detoxification, but it's not suitable for everyone. Individuals with certain medical conditions, such as diabetes or eating disorders, should avoid fasting or consult with a healthcare professional before attempting any fasting regimen. Pregnant or breastfeeding women should also refrain from fasting to ensure adequate nutrition for themselves and their babies.

For those new to fasting, starting with a short duration and gradually increasing the length of the fast can help build tolerance and confidence. Joining a fasting group or finding a fasting buddy can provide support and motivation throughout the process. Keeping a journal to track your experiences, emotions, and any physical changes can also be beneficial.

Incorporating regular fasting into your lifestyle can lead to long-term health benefits, including improved digestion, increased energy, enhanced mental clarity, and overall well-being. It's a practice that encourages mindfulness and self-awareness, allowing you to reconnect with your body and its natural rhythms.

Fasting, whether through water, juice, or fruit, is a personal journey that requires careful consideration and respect for your body's signals. It's an opportunity to give your body a break from the constant demands of digestion and allow it to focus on healing and rejuvenation. By approaching fasting with a balanced mindset and proper preparation, you can experience the profound benefits of this ancient practice and support your body's natural detoxification processes.

7, 14, and 30-Day Detox Programs

Embarking on a detox program can be a transformative experience, offering numerous benefits for your physical, mental, and emotional health. Whether you choose a 7-day, 14-day, or 30-day detox, each program has unique advantages and challenges. By following structured plans, you can maximize the detoxification process and ensure a smooth, effective journey toward better health. The 7-day detox program is an excellent starting point for those new to detoxing. It's a manageable duration that allows your body to experience the benefits of detoxification without being overwhelming. During the first two days, focus on eliminating processed foods, caffeine, and alcohol from your diet. Replace these with fresh fruits, vegetables, and plenty of water to help flush out toxins. Incorporate herbal teas that support detoxification, such as dandelion root and milk thistle.

On days three to five, you can introduce more structured meals, including green smoothies for breakfast, large salads for lunch, and vegetable-based soups for dinner. Snack on raw nuts, seeds, and fresh fruit between meals. These nutrient-dense foods support your body's natural detox processes and provide essential vitamins and minerals. It's crucial to listen to your body and adjust the plan if needed, ensuring you stay hydrated and nourished.

Days six and seven focus on reinforcing the habits you've built. Continue with the same meal structure but introduce gentle physical activity like yoga or walking to enhance circulation and further aid detoxification. By the end of the week, you should feel lighter, more energetic, and mentally clearer. The 7-day detox is a great way to kickstart healthier habits and can be repeated monthly or quarterly for ongoing benefits.

For those looking for a deeper cleanse, the 14-day detox program provides a more extended period to thoroughly eliminate toxins and reset your system. The first week follows the structure of the 7-day detox, with an emphasis on whole, unprocessed foods and plenty of hydration. As you move into the second week, you can start incorporating more specific detox practices such as intermittent fasting or juice fasting for one or two days.

Intermittent fasting involves limiting your eating to a specific window of time each day, such as an 8-hour period, and fasting for the remaining 16 hours. This practice allows your digestive system to rest and promotes cellular repair and detoxification. Juice fasting can be done by consuming only fresh vegetable and fruit juices for one or two days during the second week. This provides a nutrient boost while giving your digestive system a break.

Throughout the 14-day detox, it's important to maintain a balance between cleansing and nourishing your body. Include plenty of leafy greens, cruciferous vegetables like broccoli and cauliflower, and high-fiber foods to support digestion. Herbal teas and supplements like chlorella and spirulina can further enhance detoxification. Regular physical activity, adequate sleep, and stress management techniques such as meditation or deep breathing exercises are also crucial for a successful detox.

The 30-day detox program offers a comprehensive approach to long-term detoxification and habit formation. This program is ideal for individuals looking to make significant lifestyle changes and address chronic health issues. The first two weeks follow the guidelines of the 14-day detox, with a focus on clean eating, hydration, and gentle physical activity.

In the third week, you can introduce more advanced detox practices such as dry brushing, which helps stimulate the lymphatic system and promote the elimination of toxins through the skin. Another effective practice is hydrotherapy, which involves alternating hot and cold showers to improve circulation and support detoxification. These additional practices enhance the detox process and provide a deeper cleanse.

During the fourth week, continue with the established diet and incorporate more raw foods into your meals. Raw foods are rich in enzymes and nutrients that support detoxification and overall health. Experiment with raw salads, smoothies, and snacks like raw energy balls or dehydrated vegetable chips. This week is also a good time to focus on mental and emotional detoxification. Engage in activities that promote relaxation and stress reduction, such as journaling, spending time in nature, or practicing mindfulness. Throughout the 30-day detox, it's essential to stay attuned to your body's needs and make adjustments as necessary. Some people may experience detox symptoms such as headaches, fatigue, or skin breakouts, especially in the early stages. These symptoms are typically temporary and indicate that your body is releasing stored toxins. Ensure you get plenty of rest, stay hydrated, and seek support if needed.

A 30-day detox program not only provides a thorough cleanse but also helps establish long-lasting healthy habits. By the end of the month, you should notice significant improvements in your energy levels, digestion, skin health, and overall well-being. This program can serve as a foundation for ongoing healthy living and periodic shorter detoxes to maintain the benefits.

No matter the duration of the detox program you choose, preparation is key to success. Before starting, plan your meals, stock up on fresh produce and healthy snacks, and eliminate any temptations from your environment. Setting clear goals and intentions for your detox can also help keep you motivated and focused throughout the process. It's important to note that while detox programs can provide numerous benefits, they may not be suitable for everyone. Individuals with certain health conditions, pregnant or breastfeeding women, and those with a history of eating disorders should consult with a healthcare professional before starting any detox program. Listening to your body and respecting its limits is crucial for a safe and effective detox experience.

In conclusion, 7, 14, and 30-day detox programs offer structured approaches to cleansing your body and resetting your health. Whether you're new to detoxing or looking for a deeper cleanse, these programs provide flexibility and scalability to meet your needs. By following these guidelines and incorporating healthy habits, you can support your body's natural detoxification processes and achieve a greater sense of well-being.

Step-by-Step Instructions and Tips

Embarking on a detox program requires thoughtful planning and execution to ensure it is both effective and safe. This guide provides step-by-step instructions and practical tips to help you navigate your detox journey successfully. Whether you are undertaking a short-term detox or a longer regimen, these steps and strategies will support you in achieving optimal results.

Before starting any detox program, preparation is key. Begin by gradually reducing your intake of caffeine, sugar, alcohol, and processed foods a few days before your detox starts. This helps minimize withdrawal symptoms such as headaches and irritability, making the transition smoother. Stock up on fresh fruits, vegetables, whole grains, nuts, and seeds, and clear your pantry of temptations that could derail your detox efforts. Planning your meals and snacks ahead of time ensures that you have nutritious options readily available and reduces the likelihood of resorting to unhealthy choices.

Hydration is crucial during a detox. Aim to drink at least eight glasses of water a day to help flush out toxins and keep your body functioning optimally. Herbal teas such as dandelion, peppermint, and ginger can also support detoxification and provide additional hydration. Starting your day with a glass of warm lemon water can stimulate digestion and kickstart your metabolism.

For those engaging in a fasting-based detox, it's important to choose the type of fasting that aligns with your goals and experience level. Water fasting, where only water is consumed, is the most intensive and requires careful attention to your body's signals. Juice fasting, involving the consumption of fresh vegetable and fruit juices, offers a more balanced approach by providing essential nutrients while still allowing the digestive system to rest. Fruit fasting, which includes eating only fresh fruits, is the gentlest form and can be a good starting point for beginners.

Regardless of the fasting method chosen, listening to your body is paramount. Mild hunger, fatigue, and occasional headaches are normal as your body adjusts, but severe discomfort or dizziness may indicate that it's time to break the fast. Transitioning back to solid foods should be done gradually to avoid overwhelming your digestive system. Start with easily digestible foods like fruits and steamed vegetables, and slowly reintroduce more complex foods over the next few days.

During the detox, incorporating gentle physical activities such as walking, yoga, or stretching can enhance circulation and support the elimination of toxins. Avoid strenuous exercise, as your body may not have the energy reserves to sustain intense physical activity during a detox. Instead, focus on movements that promote relaxation and well-being.

Rest and adequate sleep are critical components of a successful detox. Your body does much of its repair and detoxification work while you sleep, so aim for seven to nine hours of quality rest each night. Creating a relaxing bedtime routine, such as reading a book or taking a warm bath, can help you wind down and improve sleep quality.

Mindfulness practices such as meditation, deep breathing, and journaling can support your detox journey by reducing stress and promoting mental clarity. Detoxification is not only a physical process but also an opportunity to clear mental and emotional clutter. Setting aside a few minutes each day for mindfulness can enhance your overall detox experience and help you stay focused on your goals.

Nutrient-dense foods play a pivotal role in supporting detoxification. Leafy greens such as spinach, kale, and arugula are rich in chlorophyll, which helps cleanse the liver and blood. Cruciferous vegetables like broccoli, cauliflower, and Brussels sprouts contain compounds that support liver function and aid in the elimination of toxins. Incorporating a variety of colorful fruits and vegetables ensures a broad spectrum of vitamins, minerals, and antioxidants to support your body's detox pathways.

Healthy fats from sources such as avocados, nuts, seeds, and olive oil provide essential fatty acids that support cell structure and function. Protein from plant-based sources like legumes, quinoa, and tempeh helps repair tissues and maintain muscle mass during detox. Fiber-rich foods such as chia seeds, flaxseeds, and whole grains promote regular bowel movements, which are essential for the elimination of toxins.

Probiotics, found in fermented foods like sauerkraut, kimchi, and kombucha, support gut health by maintaining a balanced microbiome. A healthy gut is crucial for effective detoxification, as it plays a key role in metabolizing and excreting toxins. Including these foods in your diet can enhance digestion and support overall health.

Supplements can also play a supportive role during detox. Milk thistle, known for its liver-protective properties, can help enhance liver function and promote detoxification. Spirulina and chlorella, nutrient-dense algae, bind to heavy metals and other toxins, aiding in their removal from the body. It's important to consult with a healthcare professional before adding supplements to your detox regimen to ensure they are appropriate for your individual needs.

Creating a supportive environment can significantly impact your detox success. Surround yourself with positive influences, whether it's supportive friends and family or a community of like-minded individuals. Sharing your detox journey with others can provide encouragement, accountability, and motivation. Social support is especially important during challenging moments when cravings or detox symptoms may arise.

Setting realistic goals and expectations is crucial for a successful detox. Understand that detoxification is a process, and benefits may not be immediate. Focus on the journey and the positive changes you are making for your health rather than expecting overnight results. Celebrate small victories along the way, such as increased energy levels, improved digestion, or clearer skin.

Keeping a detox journal can be a valuable tool for tracking your progress and reflecting on your experience. Record your meals, physical activity, mood, and any symptoms you experience. This can help you identify patterns, make adjustments as needed, and stay motivated. Journaling also provides an opportunity for self-reflection and mindfulness, enhancing the overall detox experience.

After completing your detox program, it's important to transition back to regular eating habits gradually. Continue to prioritize whole, nutrient-dense foods and stay hydrated. Use the insights gained during your detox to make healthier choices moving forward. Integrating elements of your detox regimen into your daily routine can help maintain the benefits and support long-term health.

In summary, a successful detox program involves careful planning, mindful practices, and a supportive environment. By following these step-by-step instructions and incorporating practical tips, you can enhance your detox experience and achieve lasting benefits for your health and well-being. Whether you're embarking on a short-term detox or a longer regimen, these strategies will support you in your journey toward a healthier, more vibrant life.

Part 5: Dr. Sebi's Treatments for Specific Diseases

Treatment for Sexually Transmitted Diseases (STDs)

Dr. Sebi's Approach

Dr. Sebi, a renowned herbalist and natural healer, developed a unique approach to treating sexually transmitted diseases (STDs) that emphasizes natural healing through diet and herbs. His methodology is rooted in the belief that maintaining an alkaline environment in the body can prevent and reverse disease. Dr. Sebi's approach focuses on removing mucus buildup, which he identified as a primary cause of many illnesses, including STDs. By detoxifying the body and restoring its natural alkaline state, Dr. Sebi believed that the body could heal itself. Central to Dr. Sebi's philosophy is the concept of cellular regeneration. He posited that by nourishing the body with natural, electric foods and avoiding acidic, processed foods, one could enhance the body's ability to regenerate healthy cells and eliminate diseased ones. This cellular regeneration is crucial in the treatment of STDs, as it involves not only the eradication of the infection but also the healing of the damaged tissues and organs.

The foundation of Dr. Sebi's treatment for STDs involves a strict adherence to an alkaline diet. This diet excludes all foods that produce acid in the body, such as meat, dairy, processed foods, and refined sugars. Instead, it promotes the consumption of alkaline foods, which include a variety of fruits, vegetables, nuts, seeds, and grains that support the body's natural pH balance. By following this diet, individuals can create an internal environment that is hostile to pathogens and conducive to healing. Another critical aspect of Dr. Sebi's approach is fasting. He advocated for periodic fasting to give the digestive system a break and allow the body to focus its energy on healing and detoxification. Fasting, according to Dr. Sebi, accelerates the elimination of toxins and mucus, which can help clear infections more rapidly. He recommended different types of fasting, including water fasting, juice fasting, and fruit fasting, depending on the individual's condition and level of experience with fasting.

In addition to diet and fasting, Dr. Sebi's treatment protocol includes the use of specific herbs known for their medicinal properties. These herbs are selected for their ability to support the immune system, reduce inflammation, and promote detoxification. By combining these herbs with an alkaline diet, Dr. Sebi aimed to strengthen the body's natural defenses and enhance its ability to fight off infections.

Detoxification is a cornerstone of Dr. Sebi's treatment for STDs. He believed that toxins and waste products accumulate in the body over time, contributing to the development and persistence of infections. By detoxifying the body, these harmful substances can be eliminated, allowing the immune system to function more effectively. Dr. Sebi's detoxification methods often involve the use of herbal teas and supplements designed to cleanse the liver, kidneys, and lymphatic system.

One of the key herbs in Dr. Sebi's protocol for treating STDs is burdock root. Known for its blood-purifying properties, burdock root helps eliminate toxins from the bloodstream, which is essential for fighting infections. It also has anti-inflammatory properties, which can help reduce the symptoms associated with STDs. Another important herb is sarsaparilla, which is rich in natural steroids that support the immune system and have anti-inflammatory effects. Sarsaparilla is also known to bind with toxins and facilitate their removal from the body. Dr. Sebi also recommended the use of chaparral, a powerful herb with antiviral properties. Chaparral has been traditionally used to treat various infections and can help inhibit the growth of viruses that cause STDs. It also supports the detoxification process by promoting the elimination of waste products through the liver and kidneys.

Sea moss, another staple in Dr. Sebi's regimen, provides a wide range of nutrients that support overall health and immune function. Rich in minerals like iodine, calcium, and potassium, sea moss helps maintain the body's alkaline state and supports the regeneration of healthy cells. It also has natural antiviral and antibacterial properties, making it an effective ally in the treatment of STDs. Incorporating these herbs into a daily routine can be done through teas, tinctures, or supplements. Dr. Sebi often recommended herbal teas made from a combination of these herbs to enhance their synergistic effects. Drinking these teas several times a day can support the body's detoxification processes and provide continuous immune support.

Dr. Sebi's approach to treating STDs also emphasizes the importance of hydration. Drinking plenty of water is crucial for flushing out toxins and maintaining overall health. Staying well-hydrated supports the kidneys in their role of filtering waste products from the blood and helps keep the body's systems functioning smoothly.While Dr. Sebi's methods focus on natural remedies and lifestyle changes, he also stressed the importance of mental and emotional health. Stress and negative emotions can weaken the immune system and impede the healing process. Therefore, he encouraged practices such as meditation, deep breathing exercises, and spending time in nature to reduce stress and promote overall well-being.

To summarize, Dr. Sebi's approach to treating STDs involves a comprehensive strategy that includes an alkaline diet, fasting, herbal supplementation, detoxification, and stress management. By addressing the root causes of illness and supporting the body's natural healing processes, this holistic method aims to eliminate infections and promote long-term health. Dr. Sebi's protocol provides a natural alternative for those seeking to treat STDs without relying on conventional pharmaceuticals, focusing instead on restoring the body's innate ability to heal itself.

Recommended Herbs and Foods

Dr. Sebi's approach to treating sexually transmitted diseases (STDs) hinges on the use of natural herbs and an alkaline diet to support the body's healing processes. By emphasizing the consumption of specific herbs and foods, his protocol aims to create an internal environment that is inhospitable to pathogens while promoting cellular regeneration and overall health. This holistic approach not only addresses the symptoms but also targets the root causes of STDs.

One of the cornerstone herbs in Dr. Sebi's regimen is burdock root. Known for its potent blood-purifying properties, burdock root helps eliminate toxins from the bloodstream, which is crucial for combating infections. It also has anti-inflammatory and antibacterial effects, which can alleviate the discomfort associated with STDs. Burdock root is often consumed as a tea or tincture, providing a continuous supply of its therapeutic benefits throughout the day. Another vital herb in Dr. Sebi's arsenal is sarsaparilla. This herb is rich in saponins, natural compounds that have been shown to bind with and eliminate toxins from the body. Sarsaparilla also supports the immune system, making it more efficient at fighting off infections. Its anti-inflammatory properties further help in reducing the symptoms of STDs, such as pain and swelling. Sarsaparilla can be taken in capsule form, as a tea, or added to smoothies for an easy and effective way to incorporate it into your daily routine.

Chaparral is another powerful herb recommended by Dr. Sebi for treating STDs. With its strong antiviral properties, chaparral helps inhibit the growth and spread of viruses responsible for infections. This herb also supports detoxification by promoting the elimination of waste products through the liver and kidneys. Consuming chaparral tea or using it in tincture form can enhance the body's ability to cleanse itself and fight off infections.

Sea moss, also known as Irish moss, plays a crucial role in Dr. Sebi's treatment protocol. This seaweed is packed with essential minerals, including iodine, potassium, and calcium, which support overall health and help maintain the body's alkaline state. Sea moss also has antiviral and antibacterial properties, making it an effective aid in fighting STDs. It can be added to smoothies, soups, or taken as a supplement to ensure a consistent intake of its beneficial nutrients.

Elderberry is another herb that Dr. Sebi recommends for its immune-boosting and antiviral properties. Elderberry has been traditionally used to treat infections and support the immune system. Its high antioxidant content helps reduce inflammation and protect cells from damage. Elderberry can be consumed as a syrup, tea, or supplement, providing versatile options for incorporating it into your diet. In addition to these specific herbs, Dr. Sebi emphasizes the importance of following an alkaline diet. This diet includes foods that help maintain the body's pH balance, making it less conducive to the survival of pathogens. Leafy greens, such as kale, spinach, and arugula, are essential components of the alkaline diet due to their high nutrient content and alkalizing properties. These greens can be consumed in salads, smoothies, or lightly steamed to retain their nutritional value.

Fruits also play a significant role in the alkaline diet. Berries, such as blueberries, strawberries, and raspberries, are rich in antioxidants and vitamins that support the immune system and promote healing. Citrus fruits, including lemons, limes, and grapefruits, are excellent sources of vitamin C, which enhances immune function and aids in detoxification. These fruits can be enjoyed fresh, in juices, or as part of various recipes to add flavor and nutritional value to your meals.

Nuts and seeds are another important component of Dr. Sebi's dietary recommendations. Almonds, chia seeds, and flaxseeds provide healthy fats, protein, and fiber, all of which support overall health and detoxification. These can be added to smoothies, salads, or consumed as snacks to ensure a balanced intake of essential nutrients.

Whole grains, such as quinoa, millet, and spelt, are preferred over refined grains in Dr. Sebi's diet. These grains are less acidic and provide essential nutrients and fiber that support digestion and detoxification. Incorporating whole grains into your diet can help maintain steady energy levels and support the body's natural cleansing processes.

Hydration is another crucial aspect of Dr. Sebi's approach. Drinking plenty of water is essential for flushing out toxins and supporting overall health. Herbal teas made from the recommended herbs, as well as fresh vegetable and fruit juices, can enhance hydration and provide additional detoxifying benefits. Coconut water is also highly recommended for its hydrating properties and nutrient content.

The preparation and consumption of these herbs and foods should be done mindfully to maximize their benefits. For instance, when preparing herbal teas, it's important to use fresh, high-quality herbs and allow them to steep properly to extract their full medicinal properties. Similarly, when consuming fruits and vegetables, opting for organic produce can reduce the intake of harmful pesticides and ensure the highest nutrient content.

Dr. Sebi also stressed the importance of avoiding certain foods that can hinder the detoxification process and exacerbate the symptoms of STDs. These include processed foods, refined sugars, dairy products, and meats, all of which can create an acidic environment in the body and promote mucus production. By eliminating these foods from your diet, you can support the body's natural ability to heal and maintain a balanced pH.

In addition to diet and herbs, Dr. Sebi advocated for a holistic approach to health that includes regular exercise, adequate rest, and stress management. Physical activity helps improve circulation and supports the elimination of toxins through sweat. Practices such as yoga, tai chi, or gentle stretching can be particularly beneficial for promoting relaxation and overall well-being.

Ensuring adequate sleep is crucial for the body's healing processes. During sleep, the body repairs tissues, regenerates cells, and detoxifies the brain. Creating a restful sleep environment and maintaining a consistent sleep schedule can support these processes and enhance overall health.

Stress management is also a vital component of Dr. Sebi's approach. Chronic stress can weaken the immune system and impair the body's ability to fight infections. Techniques such as meditation, deep breathing exercises, and spending time in nature can help reduce stress and promote a sense of calm and balance.

By integrating these recommended herbs, foods, and lifestyle practices, Dr. Sebi's approach offers a comprehensive and natural way to treat sexually transmitted diseases. This method not only targets the infections but also supports overall health and well-being, fostering a holistic healing process. Through mindful consumption of nutrient-dense foods, the use of powerful medicinal herbs, and the adoption of healthy lifestyle practices, individuals can empower their bodies to overcome infections and achieve optimal health.

Treatment for Herpes

Detailed Protocol

Herpes is a viral infection caused by the herpes simplex virus (HSV), which manifests in two main forms: HSV-1, typically associated with oral herpes, and HSV-2, primarily linked to genital herpes. Both forms of the virus can cause painful sores and blisters, and while conventional medicine asserts there is no cure, natural treatment protocols, such as those advocated by Dr. Sebi, focus on managing and reducing outbreaks through diet, herbs, and lifestyle modifications.

Dr. Sebi's protocol for treating herpes emphasizes the importance of an alkaline diet. The central tenet of this approach is to eliminate acidic foods that can contribute to inflammation and viral activity. This means avoiding processed foods, refined sugars, dairy products, and meats. Instead, the focus is on consuming fresh, alkaline-forming foods, primarily fruits, vegetables, nuts, seeds, and grains that help maintain the body's optimal pH balance. A typical day on Dr. Sebi's alkaline diet might start with a smoothie made from alkaline fruits like berries, pears, and apples, blended with leafy greens such as spinach or kale. These ingredients are rich in antioxidants, vitamins, and minerals that support the immune system and help reduce inflammation. Including a tablespoon of flaxseeds or chia seeds in the smoothie adds essential fatty acids that further enhance immune function and overall health.

For lunch, a large salad comprising a variety of raw vegetables, such as cucumbers, bell peppers, and avocados, drizzled with a lemon-tahini dressing, provides a nutrient-dense meal that supports detoxification and cellular health. The high fiber content in these vegetables aids digestion and helps the body eliminate toxins more efficiently.

Dinner could include a serving of quinoa or wild rice paired with steamed vegetables like broccoli, zucchini, and asparagus. These vegetables are not only alkaline-forming but also high in vitamins and minerals that boost the body's ability to fight viral infections. Adding a sprinkle of nutritional yeast can enhance the flavor and provide additional B vitamins, which are essential for maintaining a healthy immune system. In addition to dietary changes, Dr. Sebi's protocol includes specific herbs known for their antiviral and immune-boosting properties. One of the primary herbs recommended is burdock root. Burdock root is known for its blood-purifying properties, which help eliminate toxins from the body, thus reducing the viral load. It also has anti-inflammatory properties, which can help soothe the painful sores caused by herpes outbreaks.

Another key herb is sarsaparilla. This herb contains natural compounds that bind to toxins and facilitate their removal from the body. It is also known to boost the immune system, making it more effective at combating the herpes virus. Sarsaparilla can be consumed as a tea or in capsule form, providing a convenient way to incorporate its benefits into your daily routine.

Dr. Sebi also emphasized the use of elderberry, a powerful antiviral herb. Elderberry has been shown to inhibit the replication of viruses and reduce the duration and severity of outbreaks. It is rich in antioxidants and vitamins that support immune health, making it a valuable addition to the treatment protocol. Elderberry can be taken as a syrup, tincture, or in supplement form.

Sea moss is another essential component of Dr. Sebi's herpes treatment protocol. This seaweed is packed with essential minerals, including iodine, potassium, and calcium, which support overall health and help maintain the body's alkaline state. Sea moss also has antiviral properties and can be added to smoothies, soups, or taken as a supplement. In addition to these herbs, hydration plays a crucial role in the treatment protocol. Drinking plenty of water helps flush out toxins and supports overall bodily functions. Herbal teas made from the recommended herbs can also enhance hydration and provide additional therapeutic benefits.

Fasting is another important aspect of Dr. Sebi's approach to treating herpes. Periodic fasting allows the digestive system to rest and the body to focus on detoxification and healing. Water fasting, juice fasting, or fruit fasting can all be effective methods. For instance, a three-day water fast can kickstart the detoxification process, followed by a period of juice fasting to provide essential nutrients while continuing to cleanse the body.

Stress management is also a key component of Dr. Sebi's protocol. Stress can trigger herpes outbreaks, so incorporating relaxation techniques such as meditation, deep breathing exercises, and yoga can help manage stress levels and reduce the frequency of outbreaks. Regular physical activity, adequate sleep, and spending time in nature are also beneficial for maintaining mental and emotional well-being.

Adopting these dietary and lifestyle changes can help manage herpes more effectively. Many individuals following Dr. Sebi's protocol report fewer and less severe outbreaks, as well as an overall improvement in their health and vitality. The emphasis on natural, nutrient-dense foods and herbs, along with practices that support detoxification and immune function, provides a holistic approach to managing herpes.

It's important to note that while these natural treatments can be highly effective, individual results may vary. Consistency is key, and it may take some time to see significant improvements. Consulting with a healthcare professional before starting any new treatment regimen is also recommended, especially for individuals with underlying health conditions or those taking medications.

By following Dr. Sebi's detailed protocol for treating herpes, individuals can take a proactive approach to managing their condition. This natural, holistic method not only targets the virus itself but also supports overall health, helping the body to heal and prevent future outbreaks. Through the combination of an alkaline diet, powerful herbs, proper hydration, fasting, and stress management, individuals can work towards achieving a better quality of life and greater control over their health.

Experiences and Testimonials

The journey of managing and potentially overcoming herpes through natural methods can be deeply personal and transformative. Many individuals who have embraced Dr. Sebi's holistic approach have shared their experiences and testimonials, offering insights and encouragement to others facing similar challenges. These stories highlight the effectiveness of the protocol and the profound impact it can have on overall health and well-being.

One compelling testimonial comes from Sarah, a 32-year-old teacher who was diagnosed with HSV-2 in her mid-20s. For years, Sarah struggled with frequent and painful outbreaks that not only affected her physically but also took an emotional toll. She tried various conventional treatments, but the side effects and lack of long-term relief left her feeling frustrated and hopeless. It wasn't until she discovered Dr. Sebi's approach that she began to see significant changes.

Sarah started by transitioning to an alkaline diet, focusing on fresh fruits, vegetables, and whole grains while eliminating processed foods and sugars. She also incorporated specific herbs recommended by Dr. Sebi, such as burdock root, sarsaparilla, and elderberry. Within a few weeks, Sarah noticed a reduction in the frequency and severity of her outbreaks. Her energy levels increased, and she felt more in control of her health. Over time, her outbreaks became rare, and she experienced long periods of complete remission. Sarah credits Dr. Sebi's protocol with transforming her health and giving her a new lease on life.

Another testimonial comes from James, a 45-year-old businessman who had been living with HSV-1 for over a decade. James frequently suffered from cold sores that not only caused discomfort but also impacted his confidence, especially in professional settings. Desperate for a solution, he decided to follow Dr. Sebi's regimen. He started by incorporating sea moss into his diet, blending it into smoothies and soups. He also began drinking herbal teas made from chaparral and burdock root.

James found that within the first month, the duration and intensity of his cold sores significantly decreased. Encouraged by these results, he continued with the protocol and also introduced fasting into his routine. He practiced intermittent fasting and occasional juice fasting, which he found helped accelerate his healing process. Now, James rarely experiences cold sores, and when he does, they heal much faster than before. He feels healthier overall and more confident in his appearance and interactions.

Maria, a 28-year-old artist, shares a similar success story. Diagnosed with HSV-2, Maria experienced not only physical pain but also a profound sense of isolation and shame. Discovering Dr. Sebi's teachings offered her a sense of hope and empowerment. Maria embraced the alkaline diet, focusing on nutrient-dense foods and avoiding triggers like caffeine and alcohol. She also integrated elderberry and sea moss supplements into her daily routine.

Maria found that her body responded positively to these changes. Her immune system strengthened, and she began to have fewer outbreaks. The outbreaks that did occur were less severe and healed more quickly. Beyond the physical improvements, Maria experienced a boost in her mental and emotional well-being. She felt more in tune with her body and more confident in managing her health naturally. Maria's journey inspired her to share her story with others, helping to spread awareness about the benefits of Dr. Sebi's approach.

Alex, a 35-year-old fitness trainer, also turned to Dr. Sebi's protocol after struggling with HSV-2. As someone passionate about health and fitness, Alex was initially skeptical about the effectiveness of natural remedies. However, after experiencing limited success with conventional treatments, he decided to give it a try. Alex started by following a strict alkaline diet, incorporating plenty of green vegetables, fresh fruits, and whole grains. He also included sarsaparilla and elderberry in his regimen. To support his detoxification process, Alex practiced regular fasting, alternating between water fasting and juice fasting. He found that fasting not only helped reduce his outbreaks but also improved his overall energy and endurance. Over time, Alex experienced fewer and less severe outbreaks, and his recovery time shortened. He became a strong advocate for Dr. Sebi's methods, sharing his success with his clients and encouraging them to explore natural approaches to health. These testimonials reflect a common theme: the power of natural, holistic approaches in managing herpes. Dr. Sebi's protocol, with its emphasis on an alkaline diet, specific herbs, and lifestyle modifications, has provided many individuals with a sense of control and hope. The shared experiences of those who have followed this approach highlight the potential for significant improvements in both physical and emotional health.

The journey to healing and managing herpes through Dr. Sebi's protocol is not without its challenges. Adopting a new diet, incorporating herbal supplements, and practicing fasting require commitment and dedication. However, the stories of Sarah, James, Maria, and Alex demonstrate that with perseverance and an open mind, it is possible to achieve remarkable results. These experiences serve as a testament to the potential of natural remedies and holistic health practices in addressing chronic conditions like herpes.

For those considering Dr. Sebi's approach, it is important to start with a clear understanding of the protocol and to seek support from knowledgeable practitioners or communities. While individual results may vary, the collective experiences of those who have successfully managed their herpes through this method offer valuable insights and inspiration. By embracing the principles of natural healing, many have found relief and reclaimed their health, paving the way for a brighter, healthier future.

Treatment for HIV/AIDS

Immune Support Strategies

Treating HIV/AIDS naturally involves a comprehensive approach that focuses on bolstering the immune system, which is crucial for managing this condition. HIV attacks and weakens the immune system by targeting CD4 cells, making individuals more susceptible to infections and diseases. Therefore, supporting and strengthening the immune system is a fundamental strategy in the natural treatment of HIV/AIDS.

One of the primary ways to support the immune system is through diet. A nutrient-dense diet provides the body with the essential vitamins and minerals it needs to function optimally. Fresh fruits and vegetables, particularly those high in antioxidants, play a critical role in this process. Antioxidants help combat oxidative stress and inflammation, both of which can exacerbate the progression of HIV. Foods such as berries, leafy greens, and cruciferous vegetables are rich in vitamins A, C, and E, as well as other antioxidants that protect cells from damage.

Proteins are also essential for immune health. They are the building blocks of the body and are necessary for the repair and regeneration of tissues, including those of the immune system. Plant-based protein sources, such as legumes, nuts, seeds, and whole grains, are preferable in an immune-supportive diet. These foods provide protein without the inflammatory effects that can come from animal products. Incorporating a variety of these protein sources ensures that the body receives all the essential amino acids it needs. Healthy fats are another important component of an immune-supportive diet. Omega-3 fatty acids, found in flaxseeds, chia seeds, and walnuts, have anti-inflammatory properties that support immune function. These fats help maintain the integrity of cell membranes, ensuring that cells can communicate effectively and respond to threats. Including these fats in the diet can help reduce chronic inflammation, which is often elevated in individuals with HIV/AIDS.

In addition to diet, specific herbs and supplements can provide significant immune support. Echinacea is a well-known herb that boosts the immune system by increasing the production of white blood cells, which are crucial for fighting infections. Another beneficial herb is astragalus, which has been used in traditional Chinese medicine to enhance immune function and increase resistance to disease. Astragalus works by stimulating the production of immune cells and enhancing their activity.

Garlic is another powerful natural remedy with antiviral and immune-boosting properties. It contains allicin, a compound known for its ability to enhance the immune system and combat infections. Regular consumption of garlic can help support immune health and reduce the frequency and severity of infections in individuals with HIV/AIDS.

Medicinal mushrooms, such as reishi, shiitake, and maitake, are also valuable for immune support. These mushrooms contain beta-glucans, compounds that enhance the activity of macrophages and natural killer cells, both of which play a key role in the immune response. Incorporating these mushrooms into the diet or taking them as supplements can provide additional immune support. Probiotics are beneficial bacteria that support gut health, which is intrinsically linked to immune function. The majority of the immune system is located in the gut, so maintaining a healthy gut microbiome is crucial for overall immune health. Fermented foods, such as sauerkraut, kimchi, and kefir, are rich in probiotics and can help maintain a healthy balance of gut bacteria. Probiotic supplements can also be used to support gut health and enhance immune function. Stress management is another critical aspect of supporting the immune system. Chronic stress can weaken the immune response and accelerate the progression of HIV/AIDS. Techniques such as meditation, yoga, and deep breathing exercises can help reduce stress and promote relaxation. Regular physical activity is also beneficial for stress reduction and overall health. Engaging in activities that promote mental and emotional well-being can have a positive impact on the immune system.

Adequate sleep is essential for a healthy immune system. During sleep, the body repairs and regenerates tissues, including those of the immune system. Aim for seven to nine hours of quality sleep each night to support immune function and overall health. Creating a consistent sleep routine and a restful sleep environment can help improve sleep quality.

Hydration is another important factor in immune health. Water is essential for all bodily functions, including the immune response. Staying well-hydrated helps flush toxins from the body and supports the function of all cells, including immune cells. Aim to drink at least eight glasses of water a day, and more if you are physically active or live in a hot climate.

Regular detoxification can also support the immune system by reducing the burden of toxins that can impair immune function. Techniques such as fasting, herbal cleanses, and saunas can help remove toxins from the body and support overall health. Incorporating detoxification practices into your routine can enhance the effectiveness of the immune system. Social support is also important for individuals with HIV/AIDS. Connecting with others who understand your experience can provide emotional support and reduce feelings of isolation. Support groups, counseling, and community organizations can offer valuable resources and a sense of connection.

By integrating these immune support strategies into a comprehensive treatment plan, individuals with HIV/AIDS can enhance their immune function and improve their overall health. This holistic approach not only targets the virus itself but also supports the body's natural defenses, promoting a higher quality of life and greater resilience against infections and disease. Through a combination of a nutrient-dense diet, specific herbs and supplements, stress management, adequate sleep, hydration, detoxification, and social support, individuals can take proactive steps to manage HIV/AIDS and support their immune health.

Importance of the Alkaline Diet

The alkaline diet plays a crucial role in the treatment and management of HIV/AIDS, providing a foundation for improved health and enhanced immune function. The principle behind this diet is to maintain the body's natural pH balance, creating an environment that supports optimal cellular function and discourages the proliferation of viruses and harmful bacteria. For individuals living with HIV/AIDS, adhering to an alkaline diet can significantly impact their overall well-being and ability to manage the disease.

The body's pH level measures how acidic or alkaline it is, with a pH of 7 being neutral. Levels below 7 are acidic, and those above 7 are alkaline. The optimal pH for the human body is slightly alkaline, around 7.4. When the body becomes too acidic, it can lead to various health problems, including a weakened immune system. For someone with HIV/AIDS, maintaining an alkaline environment is vital because it helps support the immune system and reduce the viral load.

An alkaline diet primarily consists of fresh fruits, vegetables, nuts, seeds, and legumes, while avoiding acidic foods like processed foods, sugars, dairy, meat, and refined grains. This dietary approach not only supports the body's pH balance but also provides essential nutrients that are crucial for maintaining health and supporting immune function.

Fruits and vegetables are the cornerstone of the alkaline diet. They are rich in vitamins, minerals, antioxidants, and fiber, all of which are essential for supporting the immune system. Leafy greens such as spinach, kale, and Swiss chard are particularly beneficial due to their high chlorophyll content, which helps detoxify the body and support healthy blood. Chlorophyll also has anti-inflammatory properties, which can help reduce the inflammation associated with HIV/AIDS.

Cruciferous vegetables like broccoli, cauliflower, and Brussels sprouts contain compounds that support liver detoxification and boost the immune system. These vegetables are also high in fiber, which aids in digestion and helps eliminate toxins from the body. Including a variety of colorful vegetables in the diet ensures a broad spectrum of nutrients that support overall health.

Fruits such as berries, melons, and citrus fruits are excellent sources of antioxidants, which protect the body's cells from damage caused by free radicals. Antioxidants are particularly important for individuals with HIV/AIDS because they help counteract the oxidative stress that can weaken the immune system. Berries, in particular, are high in vitamins C and E, which are vital for immune health and skin integrity.

Nuts and seeds provide healthy fats, protein, and essential minerals. Almonds, chia seeds, and flaxseeds are especially beneficial due to their omega-3 fatty acid content, which has anti-inflammatory properties and supports heart health. These healthy fats are crucial for maintaining cellular health and supporting the body's immune response.

Whole grains such as quinoa, millet, and brown rice are less acidic than refined grains and provide important nutrients and fiber. These grains help maintain stable blood sugar levels and provide sustained energy, which is important for individuals managing HIV/AIDS. They also support healthy digestion, which is essential for nutrient absorption and overall health.

Hydration is another critical aspect of the alkaline diet. Drinking plenty of water helps maintain the body's pH balance and supports all bodily functions, including detoxification and immune function. Herbal teas made from alkaline-promoting herbs like nettle, dandelion, and ginger can also contribute to hydration and provide additional health benefits. These herbs have natural detoxifying properties and can support liver and kidney function, helping to eliminate toxins from the body. Incorporating alkaline-forming foods into the diet can also help manage symptoms associated with HIV/AIDS. For example, inflammation is a common issue for individuals with HIV/AIDS, and an alkaline diet rich in anti-inflammatory foods can help reduce this inflammation. By lowering inflammation, the body can better focus on repairing and regenerating cells, which is crucial for maintaining a strong immune system.

Another significant benefit of the alkaline diet is its role in supporting gut health. The majority of the immune system is located in the gut, so maintaining a healthy gut microbiome is essential for overall immune function. The high fiber content in fruits, vegetables, nuts, seeds, and whole grains supports healthy digestion and promotes the growth of beneficial gut bacteria. A balanced gut microbiome enhances nutrient absorption and helps protect against infections.

For individuals with HIV/AIDS, the alkaline diet can also help manage the side effects of antiretroviral therapy (ART). ART can cause various side effects, including gastrointestinal issues, fatigue, and nutrient deficiencies. By following an alkaline diet, individuals can support their digestive health, increase their energy levels, and ensure they are getting the nutrients they need to counteract these side effects. This dietary approach can make ART more tolerable and effective. It is important to approach the alkaline diet with balance and variety. While focusing on alkaline-forming foods, it is also essential to ensure that the diet is well-rounded and includes all necessary nutrients. Working with a nutritionist or healthcare provider can help tailor the diet to individual needs, ensuring it provides comprehensive nutritional support.

Incorporating smoothies and fresh juices made from alkaline-forming fruits and vegetables can be an effective and enjoyable way to enhance the diet. These beverages are nutrient-dense and easy to digest, making them a great option for individuals who may have compromised digestive function. Adding ingredients like spinach, kale, cucumber, berries, and citrus fruits to smoothies and juices can provide a powerful nutritional boost.

Overall, the importance of the alkaline diet in the treatment of HIV/AIDS cannot be overstated. This dietary approach supports the body's natural defenses, helps maintain a healthy pH balance, reduces inflammation, and promotes overall well-being. For individuals living with HIV/AIDS, following an alkaline diet can significantly enhance their quality of life and support their journey towards better health. By prioritizing nutrient-dense, alkaline-forming foods and maintaining proper hydration, individuals can empower themselves with a natural and effective strategy to manage their condition.

Treatment for Diabetes

Blood Sugar Control

Managing diabetes requires a comprehensive approach that focuses on controlling blood sugar levels to prevent complications and promote overall health. Blood sugar control is crucial for both type 1 and type 2 diabetes, but the strategies can vary slightly. The fundamental goal is to maintain blood glucose levels within a target range through a combination of diet, lifestyle changes, and, when necessary, medication.

Diet plays a pivotal role in blood sugar management. Consuming a balanced diet rich in whole foods helps stabilize blood sugar levels and provides the necessary nutrients to support overall health. Emphasizing low-glycemic-index (GI) foods is a key strategy. Low-GI foods are absorbed more slowly, preventing spikes in blood sugar levels. These foods include non-starchy vegetables, legumes, whole grains, and certain fruits. Incorporating these foods into daily meals helps create a steady release of glucose into the bloodstream. Non-starchy vegetables, such as leafy greens, broccoli, cauliflower, and peppers, are excellent choices for managing blood sugar. They are low in carbohydrates and high in fiber, vitamins, and minerals. Fiber is particularly important because it slows down the digestion and absorption of carbohydrates, resulting in more stable blood sugar levels. Including a variety of these vegetables in your diet can enhance blood sugar control and provide essential nutrients.

Whole grains like quinoa, barley, and oats are preferable to refined grains because they have a lower glycemic index and provide sustained energy. These grains contain more fiber and nutrients, which help regulate blood sugar levels and improve insulin sensitivity. When choosing grains, it's important to opt for those that are minimally processed to retain their nutritional benefits.

Legumes, including beans, lentils, and chickpeas, are another excellent food group for managing blood sugar. They are high in protein and fiber, which can help stabilize blood glucose levels. Protein takes longer to digest than carbohydrates, which means it can help keep you feeling full and prevent overeating, a common concern for those managing diabetes. Additionally, legumes are a great source of plant-based protein, making them a healthy alternative to animal proteins that may contain saturated fats.

Fruits with a lower glycemic index, such as berries, apples, and pears, can be enjoyed in moderation. These fruits provide essential vitamins, antioxidants, and fiber without causing significant spikes in blood sugar levels. It's beneficial to pair fruits with a source of protein or healthy fat, such as nuts or yogurt, to further moderate their impact on blood glucose.

Healthy fats, such as those found in avocados, nuts, seeds, and olive oil, are important for blood sugar management. These fats help improve insulin sensitivity and reduce inflammation, both of which are beneficial for managing diabetes. Including healthy fats in meals can help create a balanced diet that supports stable blood sugar levels.

Protein is another crucial component of a diabetes-friendly diet. It helps maintain muscle mass and supports overall health. Lean protein sources, such as chicken, turkey, fish, tofu, and tempeh, are excellent choices. Including protein in every meal can help regulate blood sugar levels and keep you feeling satisfied. In addition to dietary changes, certain herbs have been shown to help manage blood sugar levels. For example, cinnamon is known for its potential to improve insulin sensitivity and lower blood sugar levels. Adding a teaspoon of cinnamon to your diet each day, whether in smoothies, oatmeal, or tea, can provide these benefits. Similarly, fenugreek seeds contain soluble fiber, which can help control blood sugar levels. They can be soaked in water overnight and consumed in the morning or added to various dishes. Another beneficial herb is berberine, a compound found in several plants, including goldenseal and barberry. Berberine has been shown to lower blood sugar levels and improve insulin sensitivity. It is often taken in supplement form, but it's important to consult with a healthcare provider before starting any new supplement regimen.

Bitter melon is a traditional remedy used in various cultures to manage diabetes. It contains compounds that mimic insulin and help lower blood sugar levels. Bitter melon can be consumed as a juice, tea, or cooked as a vegetable. Its effectiveness varies among individuals, so it's important to monitor blood sugar levels closely when incorporating it into your diet.

Lifestyle modifications are equally important in managing diabetes. Regular physical activity helps improve insulin sensitivity and lower blood sugar levels. Aim for at least 150 minutes of moderate-intensity exercise per week, such as brisk walking, swimming, or cycling. Strength training exercises are also beneficial as they help build muscle mass, which can improve glucose metabolism.

Stress management is another critical aspect of blood sugar control. Chronic stress can lead to elevated cortisol levels, which can increase blood sugar levels. Practices such as meditation, deep breathing exercises, yoga, and spending time in nature can help reduce stress and promote overall well-being. Adequate sleep is essential for managing diabetes. Poor sleep can negatively affect blood sugar levels and insulin sensitivity. Aim for 7-9 hours of quality sleep each night and establish a consistent sleep routine to support overall health.

Hydration also plays a role in blood sugar management. Drinking plenty of water helps the kidneys flush out excess glucose through urine. Aim to drink at least eight glasses of water per day, and more if you are physically active or live in a hot climate. Monitoring blood sugar levels regularly is crucial for understanding how different foods and activities affect your blood glucose. Keeping a log of your blood sugar readings, along with your meals and activities, can help identify patterns and make necessary adjustments to your diet and lifestyle.

In conclusion, controlling blood sugar levels is fundamental for managing diabetes and preventing complications. A balanced diet rich in whole foods, low-glycemic-index foods, healthy fats, and lean proteins supports stable blood glucose levels. Incorporating specific herbs, regular physical activity, stress management, adequate sleep, and hydration further enhances blood sugar control. By adopting these strategies, individuals with diabetes can achieve better blood sugar management and improve their overall health and quality of life.

Specific Herbs and Diet

The treatment of diabetes through specific herbs and diet is a holistic approach that emphasizes the power of natural remedies and nutritious foods to manage blood sugar levels and improve overall health. This method focuses on incorporating a variety of herbs known for their antidiabetic properties and adopting a diet rich in whole, unprocessed foods that support stable blood glucose levels.

One of the most effective herbs for managing diabetes is fenugreek. Fenugreek seeds are high in soluble fiber, which helps slow down the digestion and absorption of carbohydrates, resulting in lower blood sugar levels. These seeds can be soaked overnight and consumed with water in the morning or added to various dishes. The compounds in fenugreek not only help regulate blood sugar but also improve insulin sensitivity, making it easier for the body to use insulin effectively.

Another powerful herb is bitter melon, which has been used traditionally to manage diabetes. Bitter melon contains active compounds that mimic insulin and help reduce blood glucose levels. This herb can be consumed as a juice, tea, or cooked as a vegetable. While the taste may be bitter, the benefits for blood sugar control are significant. Regular consumption of bitter melon can lead to noticeable improvements in blood glucose management.

Cinnamon is another well-known spice with antidiabetic properties. It has been shown to lower blood sugar levels by improving insulin sensitivity and enhancing glucose uptake by cells. Adding cinnamon to your diet can be as simple as sprinkling it on oatmeal, yogurt, or smoothies. Its pleasant flavor makes it an easy addition to many dishes, and its health benefits make it a valuable component of a diabetes management plan.

Berberine, a compound found in several plants, including goldenseal and barberry, is also highly effective in managing diabetes. Berberine helps lower blood sugar levels by activating an enzyme called AMP-activated protein kinase (AMPK), which plays a role in regulating metabolism. This compound also improves insulin sensitivity and reduces the production of glucose in the liver. Berberine supplements are widely available, but it is important to consult with a healthcare provider before starting any new supplement.

Turmeric, with its active compound curcumin, is another valuable herb for diabetes management. Curcumin has anti-inflammatory and antioxidant properties that can help reduce inflammation and oxidative stress, both of which are associated with diabetes. Incorporating turmeric into your diet can be done by adding it to curries, soups, or smoothies. Turmeric supplements are also available for those who prefer a more concentrated dose.

The diet for managing diabetes should focus on whole, unprocessed foods that provide a steady release of energy without causing spikes in blood sugar levels. Non-starchy vegetables, such as leafy greens, broccoli, cauliflower, and peppers, are excellent choices because they are low in carbohydrates and high in fiber, vitamins, and minerals. Fiber is particularly important for blood sugar control because it slows down the absorption of sugar and helps maintain stable glucose levels.

Whole grains, such as quinoa, barley, and brown rice, are preferable to refined grains because they have a lower glycemic index and provide sustained energy. These grains are rich in fiber and nutrients that help regulate blood sugar levels and improve insulin sensitivity. Including a variety of whole grains in your diet can help maintain stable blood glucose levels and provide essential nutrients.

Legumes, including beans, lentils, and chickpeas, are another important component of a diabetes-friendly diet. They are high in protein and fiber, which can help stabilize blood glucose levels. Protein takes longer to digest than carbohydrates, which means it can help keep you feeling full and prevent overeating. Additionally, legumes are a great source of plant-based protein, making them a healthy alternative to animal proteins that may contain saturated fats.

Healthy fats, such as those found in avocados, nuts, seeds, and olive oil, are essential for blood sugar management. These fats help improve insulin sensitivity and reduce inflammation, both of which are beneficial for managing diabetes. Including healthy fats in meals can help create a balanced diet that supports stable blood sugar levels.

Protein is another crucial component of a diabetes-friendly diet. It helps maintain muscle mass and supports overall health. Lean protein sources, such as chicken, turkey, fish, tofu, and tempeh, are excellent choices. Including protein in every meal can help regulate blood sugar levels and keep you feeling satisfied.

Incorporating these dietary changes along with specific herbs can significantly enhance diabetes management. It is important to approach this process with consistency and dedication, as the benefits of a healthy diet and herbal supplementation are most evident when maintained over time.

In addition to dietary changes and herbs, regular physical activity plays a critical role in managing diabetes. Exercise helps improve insulin sensitivity and lower blood sugar levels. Aim for at least 150 minutes of moderate-intensity exercise per week, such as brisk walking, swimming, or cycling. Strength training exercises are also beneficial as they help build muscle mass, which can improve glucose metabolism.

Stress management is another essential aspect of diabetes management. Chronic stress can lead to elevated cortisol levels, which can increase blood sugar levels. Practices such as meditation, yoga, and deep breathing exercises can help reduce stress and promote relaxation. Regular physical activity is also beneficial for stress reduction and overall health.

Adequate sleep is essential for managing diabetes. Poor sleep can negatively affect blood sugar levels and insulin sensitivity. Aim for 7-9 hours of quality sleep each night and establish a consistent sleep routine to support overall health.

Hydration is also important for blood sugar management. Drinking plenty of water helps the kidneys flush out excess glucose through urine. Aim to drink at least eight glasses of water per day, and more if you are physically active or live in a hot climate.

Monitoring blood sugar levels regularly is crucial for understanding how different foods and activities affect your blood glucose. Keeping a log of your blood sugar readings, along with your meals and activities, can help identify patterns and make necessary adjustments to your diet and lifestyle.

In summary, the treatment of diabetes through specific herbs and diet involves a comprehensive approach that emphasizes the power of natural remedies and nutritious foods to manage blood sugar levels and improve overall health. Incorporating herbs such as fenugreek, bitter melon, cinnamon, berberine, and turmeric into your daily routine, along with a diet rich in whole, unprocessed foods, can significantly enhance diabetes management. By adopting these strategies, individuals with diabetes can achieve better blood sugar control and improve their overall health and quality of life.

Treatment for Lupus

Inflammation Reduction

Lupus, an autoimmune disease, causes the immune system to mistakenly attack healthy tissues, leading to inflammation, pain, and damage to various parts of the body. Managing lupus effectively requires a comprehensive approach, with inflammation reduction being a crucial component of treatment. Reducing inflammation not only alleviates symptoms but also helps prevent long-term tissue damage and improves overall quality of life.

One of the primary strategies for reducing inflammation in lupus patients is through diet. A diet rich in anti-inflammatory foods can significantly decrease inflammation and support overall health. Fresh fruits and vegetables, particularly those high in antioxidants, are essential. Antioxidants combat oxidative stress and reduce inflammation at the cellular level. Berries, such as blueberries, strawberries, and blackberries, are excellent sources of antioxidants. These fruits can be easily incorporated into the diet through smoothies, salads, or as snacks. Leafy greens like spinach, kale, and Swiss chard are packed with vitamins, minerals, and phytochemicals that have anti-inflammatory properties. These greens can be included in salads, smoothies, or lightly sautéed as a side dish. Cruciferous vegetables, such as broccoli, cauliflower, and Brussels sprouts, are also beneficial due to their high content of sulforaphane, a compound known for its potent anti-inflammatory effects.

Healthy fats are another vital component of an anti-inflammatory diet. Omega-3 fatty acids, found in fatty fish like salmon, mackerel, and sardines, as well as in flaxseeds, chia seeds, and walnuts, have been shown to reduce inflammation. These fats help balance the body's inflammatory response and can alleviate the joint pain and stiffness often associated with lupus. Including these sources of omega-3s in your diet regularly can provide significant benefits.

In contrast, it is important to avoid or limit foods that can increase inflammation. Processed foods, refined sugars, and trans fats are known to exacerbate inflammation and should be minimized. Instead, focus on whole, unprocessed foods that nourish the body and support a healthy immune response. Herbs and spices are also powerful allies in reducing inflammation. Turmeric, with its active compound curcumin, is one of the most effective natural anti-inflammatory agents. Curcumin inhibits several molecules that play a role in inflammation. Adding turmeric to your diet can be as simple as sprinkling it on roasted vegetables, mixing it into soups, or blending it into smoothies. For a more potent dose, turmeric supplements are available, but it is important to consult with a healthcare provider before starting any new supplement. Ginger is another spice with strong anti-inflammatory properties. It contains compounds called gingerols and shogaols that help reduce inflammation and pain. Fresh ginger can be grated into teas, smoothies, and stir-fries, or ginger supplements can be taken to achieve these benefits.

Bromelain, an enzyme found in pineapples, is known for its anti-inflammatory and pain-relieving properties. Bromelain can help reduce the inflammation and swelling that are common in lupus. While fresh pineapple is a good source, bromelain supplements are available for those who need a higher dose.

In addition to diet, lifestyle changes play a crucial role in managing inflammation in lupus. Regular physical activity helps reduce inflammation and improve overall health. Low-impact exercises such as walking, swimming, and yoga are particularly beneficial for lupus patients as they help maintain joint flexibility and reduce stiffness without putting too much strain on the body. Consistency is key, so finding enjoyable activities that can be done regularly is important.

Stress management is another critical factor. Chronic stress can exacerbate inflammation and trigger lupus flare-ups. Techniques such as mindfulness meditation, deep breathing exercises, and progressive muscle relaxation can help manage stress and reduce its impact on the body. Engaging in hobbies, spending time in nature, and connecting with supportive friends and family can also contribute to stress reduction. Adequate sleep is essential for reducing inflammation and allowing the body to repair itself. Poor sleep can increase inflammation and make lupus symptoms worse. Establishing a regular sleep routine, creating a restful sleep environment, and practicing good sleep hygiene can help improve sleep quality. Aim for seven to nine hours of sleep per night to support overall health.

Hydration is another important aspect of inflammation reduction. Staying well-hydrated helps flush toxins from the body and supports overall health. Drinking plenty of water throughout the day is crucial. Herbal teas, such as green tea and chamomile, can also provide hydration along with additional anti-inflammatory benefits. Supplements can also play a role in reducing inflammation in lupus patients. Vitamin D, for example, has been shown to have anti-inflammatory effects and may help modulate the immune system. Many people with lupus are deficient in vitamin D, so supplementation can be beneficial. Omega-3 supplements can also be used to ensure an adequate intake of these essential fatty acids.

Probiotics are another supplement to consider. A healthy gut microbiome is crucial for overall health and can influence the body's inflammatory response. Probiotic supplements can help maintain a healthy balance of gut bacteria, which in turn can help reduce inflammation.

Incorporating these dietary and lifestyle changes can significantly reduce inflammation and improve the quality of life for individuals with lupus. It's important to approach these changes gradually and consistently, making adjustments as needed based on individual responses and needs. Working with a healthcare provider or nutritionist can help tailor these strategies to each individual's specific situation.

By focusing on anti-inflammatory foods, beneficial herbs and spices, regular physical activity, stress management, adequate sleep, and appropriate supplementation, individuals with lupus can effectively manage inflammation and support their overall health. This comprehensive approach not only addresses the symptoms of lupus but also promotes a healthier, more balanced lifestyle.

Nutrition and Supplements

Managing lupus through nutrition and supplements involves adopting a holistic approach that emphasizes the consumption of anti-inflammatory foods and specific nutrients to support overall health and reduce the symptoms associated with this autoimmune disease. The goal is to nourish the body in a way that helps modulate the immune system, minimize inflammation, and promote healing.

One of the foundational elements of a lupus-friendly diet is the inclusion of anti-inflammatory foods. These foods help to combat the chronic inflammation that is characteristic of lupus. Fresh fruits and vegetables are at the top of the list. Leafy greens such as spinach, kale, and Swiss chard are particularly beneficial due to their high content of vitamins, minerals, and antioxidants. These greens help to reduce oxidative stress and inflammation in the body.

Berries are another excellent choice for individuals with lupus. Blueberries, strawberries, raspberries, and blackberries are packed with antioxidants and phytonutrients that support immune function and reduce inflammation. Adding a variety of berries to your diet can provide a significant boost to your overall health and help manage lupus symptoms more effectively.

Fatty fish, such as salmon, mackerel, sardines, and trout, are rich in omega-3 fatty acids, which have powerful anti-inflammatory properties. Omega-3s help reduce the production of inflammatory cytokines and support overall cardiovascular health, which is often a concern for those with lupus. Including fatty fish in your diet several times a week can provide these beneficial fats and help keep inflammation in check.

Nuts and seeds, including walnuts, flaxseeds, and chia seeds, are also excellent sources of omega-3 fatty acids. They can be easily incorporated into meals or snacks and provide a plant-based source of these essential fats. Additionally, nuts and seeds offer a good amount of fiber, protein, and other vital nutrients that support overall health.

Whole grains, such as quinoa, brown rice, and oats, are preferable to refined grains because they have a lower glycemic index and provide more nutrients. Whole grains help maintain stable blood sugar levels and reduce inflammation. They are also rich in fiber, which supports healthy digestion and can help manage weight, another important factor for those with lupus.

Olive oil, particularly extra virgin olive oil, is another key component of an anti-inflammatory diet. It contains oleocanthal, a compound with anti-inflammatory properties similar to those of non-steroidal anti-inflammatory drugs (NSAIDs). Using olive oil as your primary cooking oil and for dressings can help reduce inflammation and support heart health.

Turmeric is a spice that has gained recognition for its anti-inflammatory and antioxidant properties, largely due to its active compound curcumin. Including turmeric in your diet can help reduce inflammation and support immune function. Turmeric can be added to curries, soups, smoothies, or taken as a supplement for a more concentrated dose.

Ginger is another spice with potent anti-inflammatory effects. It has been used for centuries in traditional medicine to treat various inflammatory conditions. Fresh ginger can be grated into teas, smoothies, or cooked dishes to provide these benefits. Ginger supplements are also available for those who prefer a more consistent intake.

Green tea is a beverage that offers numerous health benefits, including anti-inflammatory effects. It contains polyphenols, which are antioxidants that help reduce inflammation and protect against cellular damage. Drinking green tea regularly can support overall health and provide a calming effect, which can be beneficial for managing stress—a common trigger for lupus flares.

In addition to these dietary changes, certain supplements can play a crucial role in managing lupus. Vitamin D is particularly important, as many individuals with lupus are deficient in this nutrient. Vitamin D supports immune function and helps reduce the risk of osteoporosis, which can be a concern for those with lupus. Regularly monitoring vitamin D levels and supplementing as needed can help maintain adequate levels and support overall health.

Omega-3 supplements, derived from fish oil or algae oil, can be beneficial for those who may not get enough through their diet. These supplements provide a concentrated source of omega-3 fatty acids, helping to reduce inflammation and support cardiovascular health.

Probiotics are another valuable supplement for individuals with lupus. They support gut health, which is closely linked to immune function. A healthy gut microbiome can help modulate the immune system and reduce inflammation. Including probiotic-rich foods like yogurt, kefir, sauerkraut, and kimchi in your diet, or taking a high-quality probiotic supplement, can support gut health and overall well-being.

Magnesium is a mineral that supports muscle and nerve function, and it can also help reduce inflammation. Many people with lupus experience muscle pain and cramps, and ensuring adequate magnesium intake can help alleviate these symptoms. Foods rich in magnesium include dark leafy greens, nuts, seeds, and whole grains. Magnesium supplements are also available for those who need additional support.

Selenium is another important mineral with antioxidant properties that support immune function and reduce inflammation. Brazil nuts are an excellent source of selenium, and just one or two nuts per day can provide the recommended daily intake. Selenium supplements can also be used, but it is important not to exceed the recommended dose, as high levels of selenium can be toxic.

Coenzyme Q10 (CoQ10) is a powerful antioxidant that supports cellular energy production and reduces oxidative stress. CoQ10 levels can be depleted by certain medications commonly used to treat lupus, such as statins. Supplementing with CoQ10 can help restore these levels and support overall health. CoQ10 supplements are widely available and can be taken daily to provide these benefits.

While nutrition and supplements play a crucial role in managing lupus, it is essential to approach treatment with a comprehensive plan that includes regular medical care and monitoring. Working with a healthcare provider to tailor a diet and supplement regimen to your specific needs can help optimize your health and manage lupus symptoms more effectively.

Incorporating these dietary changes and supplements into your daily routine can help reduce inflammation, support immune function, and improve overall health. By focusing on nutrient-dense, anti-inflammatory foods and strategic supplementation, individuals with lupus can take proactive steps to manage their condition and enhance their quality of life.

Treatment for Hair Loss

Nutrition for Scalp Health

Treating hair loss effectively involves a comprehensive approach that addresses the underlying causes, one of which is often poor nutrition. Proper nutrition plays a crucial role in maintaining a healthy scalp and promoting hair growth. By focusing on nutrient-rich foods that support scalp health, you can create an optimal environment for hair follicles to thrive and reduce hair loss. A balanced diet that includes a variety of vitamins, minerals, and other essential nutrients is key to promoting scalp health and preventing hair loss. One of the most important nutrients for hair health is protein. Hair is primarily made up of keratin, a type of protein, so consuming adequate amounts of protein is essential for hair growth and strength. Good sources of protein include lean meats, fish, eggs, beans, and nuts. Ensuring that your diet contains sufficient protein helps maintain the structural integrity of hair follicles and encourages healthy hair growth.

Iron is another critical nutrient for scalp health and hair growth. Iron deficiency can lead to anemia, a condition that reduces the oxygen supply to hair follicles, leading to hair thinning and loss. Foods rich in iron include red meat, poultry, fish, lentils, spinach, and fortified cereals. Combining iron-rich foods with vitamin C-rich foods, such as citrus fruits, strawberries, and bell peppers, can enhance iron absorption and maximize its benefits for hair health.

Zinc is a mineral that plays a vital role in maintaining a healthy scalp. It helps regulate the production of sebum, the natural oil produced by sebaceous glands, which keeps the scalp moisturized and prevents dryness and flakiness. Foods high in zinc include oysters, beef, pumpkin seeds, and chickpeas. Adequate zinc intake can help prevent dandruff and maintain a healthy scalp environment conducive to hair growth.

Omega-3 fatty acids are essential for maintaining the health of the scalp and promoting hair growth. These healthy fats help reduce inflammation, which can affect the health of hair follicles. Omega-3 fatty acids also help keep the scalp hydrated and support the production of natural oils. Sources of omega-3s include fatty fish such as salmon, mackerel, and sardines, as well as flaxseeds, chia seeds, and walnuts. Including these foods in your diet can help improve scalp health and reduce hair loss.

Biotin, also known as vitamin B7, is a water-soluble vitamin that supports the health of hair, skin, and nails. Biotin deficiency can lead to hair thinning and hair loss. Foods rich in biotin include eggs, almonds, sweet potatoes, and avocados. Including biotin-rich foods in your diet can help strengthen hair and promote growth. Biotin supplements are also available for those who need an additional boost.

Vitamin A is essential for cell growth, including the cells in the scalp and hair follicles. It also helps the scalp produce sebum, which keeps hair moisturized and healthy. Foods high in vitamin A include sweet potatoes, carrots, spinach, and kale. However, it is important not to consume excessive amounts of vitamin A, as too much can lead to toxicity and potentially contribute to hair loss.

Vitamin E is another important nutrient for hair health. It has antioxidant properties that help protect hair follicles from oxidative damage. Vitamin E also supports circulation, which helps deliver nutrients to the scalp and hair follicles. Foods rich in vitamin E include almonds, sunflower seeds, spinach, and avocados. Including these foods in your diet can help maintain healthy hair and reduce hair loss.

Vitamin D is crucial for maintaining healthy hair follicles. A deficiency in vitamin D has been linked to alopecia, a condition that causes hair thinning and loss. The body produces vitamin D when exposed to sunlight, but it can also be obtained from dietary sources such as fatty fish, fortified dairy products, and egg yolks. For those who have limited sun exposure, vitamin D supplements may be beneficial.

In addition to these specific nutrients, maintaining overall hydration is essential for scalp health. Drinking plenty of water helps keep the scalp and hair hydrated, which is important for preventing dryness and breakage. Staying well-hydrated supports the health of every cell in the body, including those in the scalp and hair follicles. Incorporating these nutrient-rich foods into your daily diet can create a strong foundation for healthy hair growth and reduce hair loss. It is important to maintain a balanced diet that includes a variety of these nutrients to ensure that your scalp and hair follicles receive all the support they need. While proper nutrition is fundamental for scalp health, it is also important to consider the impact of lifestyle factors on hair loss. Stress, for example, can have a significant impact on hair health. Chronic stress can lead to a condition called telogen effluvium, where hair prematurely enters the resting phase and falls out. Managing stress through practices such as meditation, yoga, and regular physical activity can help reduce its impact on hair health. Getting adequate sleep is another important factor in maintaining a healthy scalp and promoting hair growth. During sleep, the body undergoes various repair and regeneration processes, including those that affect hair follicles. Aim for seven to nine hours of quality sleep each night to support overall health and well-being. Avoiding excessive heat styling and harsh chemical treatments can also help prevent hair damage and loss. Heat and chemicals can weaken the hair shaft and lead to breakage. Using gentle hair care products and minimizing the use of heat styling tools can help maintain the integrity of the hair and scalp.

In summary, nutrition plays a crucial role in maintaining a healthy scalp and promoting hair growth. By incorporating a variety of nutrient-rich foods into your diet, you can support the health of your hair follicles and reduce hair loss. Combining a balanced diet with healthy lifestyle practices can help create an optimal environment for hair growth and improve overall hair health. This holistic approach to hair loss treatment addresses the underlying causes and provides a sustainable solution for maintaining healthy hair.

Herbal Remedies

In addition to proper nutrition, herbal remedies offer a natural and effective way to treat hair loss. These remedies have been used for centuries across various cultures to promote hair growth and improve scalp health. By incorporating specific herbs into your hair care routine, you can enhance the vitality of your hair and reduce hair loss.

One of the most well-known herbs for hair health is rosemary. Rosemary is rich in antioxidants and has anti-inflammatory properties that can improve scalp circulation and stimulate hair growth. It can also help prevent hair follicles from being starved of blood supply, leading to hair loss. Rosemary oil can be massaged into the scalp to enhance blood flow and promote hair growth. To use, mix a few drops of rosemary essential oil with a carrier oil like coconut or olive oil and massage it into the scalp. Leave it on for at least 30 minutes before washing it out. Regular use can result in thicker, healthier hair. Another beneficial herb is aloe vera. Aloe vera has soothing and moisturizing properties that can alleviate scalp irritation and create a healthy environment for hair growth. It contains enzymes that repair dead skin cells on the scalp and promote hair growth. Aloe vera gel can be applied directly to the scalp and hair. Leave it on for about an hour before rinsing it off with a mild shampoo. Using aloe vera regularly can help reduce dandruff, unblock hair follicles that may be blocked by excess oil, and restore the natural pH balance of the scalp.

Ginseng is a powerful herb that has been traditionally used in Asian medicine to promote hair growth. It contains ginsenosides, which are active components that can enhance hair strength and reduce hair loss. Ginseng improves the proliferation of dermal papilla cells in the scalp, which play a key role in the regulation of hair growth. Ginseng extract can be taken as a supplement or used topically in the form of ginseng-infused hair products. Regular use can revitalize hair follicles and promote healthier hair. Horsetail is another herb known for its benefits to hair health. It is rich in silica, a mineral that strengthens hair strands, improves hair texture, and reduces hair breakage. Horsetail also contains antioxidants and anti-inflammatory properties that support scalp health. Horsetail extract can be taken as a supplement, or horsetail tea can be used as a hair rinse. To make a hair rinse, steep horsetail in boiling water, let it cool, and then pour it over your hair after shampooing. Leave it on for a few minutes before rinsing it out. This can help strengthen hair and enhance its natural shine.

Saw palmetto is an herb that has been studied for its potential to reduce hair loss, particularly in cases of androgenetic alopecia (pattern baldness). It works by inhibiting the conversion of testosterone to dihydrotestosterone (DHT), a hormone that can cause hair follicles to shrink and lead to hair loss. Saw palmetto can be taken as an oral supplement or used topically in hair products. Regular use may help slow down hair loss and promote hair growth.

Peppermint oil is another effective remedy for promoting hair growth. Peppermint oil has cooling and soothing properties that can increase blood circulation to the scalp and stimulate hair follicles. It also has antimicrobial properties that can help maintain a healthy scalp. To use peppermint oil, mix a few drops with a carrier oil and massage it into the scalp. Leave it on for at least 30 minutes before washing it out. Regular application can help improve hair density and encourage new hair growth.

Lavender oil is known for its calming and soothing properties, but it also has benefits for hair health. Lavender oil can improve scalp circulation, promote hair growth, and reduce hair loss. It also has antimicrobial properties that can help prevent dandruff and other scalp infections. To use lavender oil, mix a few drops with a carrier oil and massage it into the scalp. Leave it on for at least 30 minutes before rinsing it out. Using lavender oil regularly can help maintain a healthy scalp and promote thicker, healthier hair.

Neem oil is derived from the neem tree and is known for its antifungal, antibacterial, and anti-inflammatory properties. Neem oil can help treat scalp conditions that contribute to hair loss, such as dandruff and fungal infections. It also helps improve hair strength and shine. Neem oil can be applied directly to the scalp and hair. To use, warm a small amount of neem oil and massage it into the scalp. Leave it on for at least 30 minutes before washing it out with a mild shampoo. Regular use can help improve scalp health and reduce hair loss.

Nettle, or stinging nettle, is a herb that has been used for centuries to promote hair growth and reduce hair loss. It contains silica and sulfur, which help make hair shinier and healthier. Nettle also helps in blocking DHT, a hormone that can cause hair loss. Nettle tea can be consumed to provide internal benefits, or nettle extract can be applied directly to the scalp. To use nettle as a hair rinse, steep nettle leaves in boiling water, let it cool, and pour it over your hair after shampooing. Leave it on for a few minutes before rinsing it out.

Bhringraj, also known as false daisy, is an herb used in Ayurvedic medicine to promote hair growth and reduce hair loss. It is believed to improve blood circulation to the scalp and stimulate hair follicles. Bhringraj oil can be applied to the scalp and hair. To use, warm the oil and massage it into the scalp. Leave it on for at least 30 minutes before washing it out. Regular use of Bhringraj oil can help strengthen hair roots and promote healthy hair growth.

These herbal remedies, when combined with a nutritious diet, can create a comprehensive approach to treating hair loss. By addressing both internal and external factors that contribute to hair loss, you can promote a healthy scalp environment and encourage hair growth. Consistent use of these herbal remedies can provide noticeable improvements in hair health and reduce hair loss over time.

Treatment for Cancer

Dr. Sebi's Unconventional Approach

Dr. Sebi's approach to treating cancer is rooted in his belief that disease results from an overaccumulation of mucus and toxins in the body, which creates an acidic environment conducive to disease. His unconventional methods focus on detoxifying the body, restoring its natural alkaline state, and using specific herbs and foods to promote healing and enhance the immune system. This holistic strategy aims to address the underlying causes of cancer, rather than just treating its symptoms.

Central to Dr. Sebi's approach is the alkaline diet, which emphasizes the consumption of natural, plant-based foods that help maintain the body's pH balance. He believed that an acidic body environment allows cancer cells to thrive, while an alkaline environment inhibits their growth. The diet excludes all processed foods, meats, dairy, and refined sugars, focusing instead on fruits, vegetables, nuts, seeds, and grains that are alkaline-forming. This dietary shift is designed to cleanse the body of toxins and reduce inflammation, which can contribute to cancer progression.

One of the key components of the alkaline diet is the consumption of raw fruits and vegetables, which are rich in vitamins, minerals, and antioxidants. These nutrients support the body's natural detoxification processes and strengthen the immune system. Leafy greens such as kale, spinach, and arugula are particularly emphasized for their high chlorophyll content, which helps cleanse the blood and tissues. Berries, known for their high antioxidant content, are also a staple in the diet, as they help neutralize free radicals and protect cells from damage.

Dr. Sebi also recommended the use of specific herbs known for their detoxifying and healing properties. Burdock root is one such herb, prized for its ability to purify the blood and support liver function. The liver is a critical organ in the detoxification process, and by enhancing its function, burdock root helps remove toxins more efficiently from the body. This detoxification is crucial in creating an internal environment that is less hospitable to cancer cells.

Sarsaparilla is another herb frequently used in Dr. Sebi's protocol. It contains natural compounds that bind to toxins and facilitate their elimination from the body. Sarsaparilla is also known for its anti-inflammatory properties, which can help reduce the chronic inflammation often associated with cancer. By reducing inflammation, sarsaparilla supports the body's ability to heal and regenerate healthy cells.

Sea moss, a type of seaweed, is another important component of Dr. Sebi's treatment regimen. Sea moss is rich in iodine, calcium, potassium, and other essential minerals that support overall health and cellular function. It also has natural antiviral and antibacterial properties, which can help protect the body from infections that might complicate cancer treatment. Incorporating sea moss into the diet can provide a broad range of nutrients that support the immune system and promote healing. Fasting is another significant aspect of Dr. Sebi's approach. He believed that fasting helps the body focus its energy on healing and detoxification rather than digestion. By giving the digestive system a break, fasting allows the body to cleanse itself more effectively. There are different types of fasting, including water fasting, juice fasting, and fruit fasting, each with its own benefits. Water fasting, for example, can induce a state of autophagy, where the body breaks down and recycles damaged cells, potentially including cancer cells.

Dr. Sebi's unconventional approach also includes the use of natural supplements to support overall health and the immune system. One such supplement is spirulina, a type of blue-green algae that is rich in protein, vitamins, and minerals. Spirulina has been shown to have immune-boosting and anti-inflammatory effects, making it a valuable addition to the diet of someone undergoing cancer treatment. Another supplement often recommended is chlorella, another type of algae known for its detoxifying properties. Chlorella binds to heavy metals and other toxins, helping to remove them from the body. It also supports immune function and provides essential nutrients that can help the body heal.

Dr. Sebi's approach to cancer treatment is not solely focused on diet and herbs; it also emphasizes the importance of mental and emotional health. Stress and negative emotions can weaken the immune system and hinder the body's ability to heal. Practices such as meditation, deep breathing exercises, and spending time in nature are encouraged to reduce stress and promote a positive mindset. Creating a supportive environment and maintaining a positive outlook are considered essential components of the healing process.

His methods have been met with both support and skepticism. While many individuals have reported positive outcomes and improvements in their health after following his protocols, it is important to note that scientific evidence supporting the efficacy of these treatments is limited. Cancer is a complex disease, and while natural and holistic approaches can provide significant benefits, they should be considered as complementary to conventional medical treatments.

Case studies and personal testimonials from individuals who have followed Dr. Sebi's approach often highlight remarkable recoveries and improvements in quality of life. These stories frequently mention increased energy levels, reduced pain, and the shrinking of tumors. While these anecdotes provide hope and encouragement, it is essential for individuals to consult with healthcare professionals before making significant changes to their treatment plans.

In summary, Dr. Sebi's unconventional approach to cancer treatment focuses on detoxifying the body, maintaining an alkaline diet, and using specific herbs and natural supplements to support the immune system and promote healing. This holistic method addresses the underlying causes of disease and emphasizes the importance of overall health and well-being. While the effectiveness of these treatments varies among individuals, many have found relief and improvement in their condition through this natural approach. As with any treatment plan, it is crucial to consider these methods as part of a comprehensive strategy that includes guidance from healthcare professionals.

Case Studies and Results

Dr. Sebi's unconventional approach to cancer treatment has garnered significant attention and curiosity. His methodology focuses on holistic healing, emphasizing an alkaline diet and natural herbs to combat cancer's root causes. While his approach diverges from traditional medical treatments, numerous individuals have reported remarkable improvements in their health after following his protocol. This section delves into several case studies and the results experienced by those who have embraced Dr. Sebi's treatment.

One of the most notable case studies involves a patient named Maria, a 55-year-old woman diagnosed with stage IV breast cancer. After undergoing conventional treatments such as chemotherapy and radiation, Maria experienced severe side effects and minimal improvement. Frustrated and seeking alternatives, she turned to Dr. Sebi's approach. Maria adopted a strict alkaline diet, eliminating all acidic foods and focusing on consuming fresh fruits, vegetables, and herbal teas. She also incorporated key herbs recommended by Dr. Sebi, including burdock root, sarsaparilla, and sea moss.

Within a few months, Maria noticed significant changes in her health. Her energy levels increased, and the side effects she experienced from previous treatments began to subside. Regular medical check-ups revealed a reduction in tumor size and an improvement in her overall condition. Maria's case demonstrates how an alkaline diet and specific herbs can support the body's natural healing processes, offering hope to those seeking alternative treatments for cancer.

Another compelling case involves James, a 48-year-old man diagnosed with colon cancer. James was skeptical about abandoning conventional treatments but decided to complement his chemotherapy with Dr. Sebi's dietary recommendations. He started consuming more alkaline foods, such as leafy greens, berries, and whole grains, while eliminating processed foods, red meat, and sugars. Additionally, he used herbs like bladderwrack and dandelion root to support detoxification and overall health.

James reported feeling more resilient and less fatigued during his chemotherapy sessions. Blood tests indicated that his immune system remained robust despite the aggressive treatment, which his doctors attributed to his improved diet and herbal supplementation. Over time, scans showed a decrease in tumor size, and James entered remission. His experience highlights the potential benefits of integrating holistic dietary changes with conventional cancer treatments.

Sarah, a 60-year-old woman with ovarian cancer, provides another insightful case study. After her diagnosis, Sarah faced limited treatment options due to the advanced stage of her cancer. She decided to fully commit to Dr. Sebi's approach, hoping to improve her quality of life and possibly extend her survival. Sarah adhered to a stringent alkaline diet, avoiding all acidic foods and beverages. She also included herbs like yellow dock, chaparral, and nettle in her regimen.

Sarah experienced significant pain relief and increased vitality. Her regular scans showed stabilization of the cancer, with no further progression. Although her cancer was not cured, Sarah's quality of life improved dramatically, allowing her to spend more meaningful time with her family. Her case underscores the importance of quality of life considerations in cancer treatment and the potential for alternative approaches to provide relief and stability.

Another noteworthy case is that of Robert, a 52-year-old man with prostate cancer. Robert's treatment journey began with standard medical interventions, but he sought additional support through Dr. Sebi's methods. He adopted the alkaline diet and incorporated herbs like elderberry, ginger, and Irish moss. Robert's primary goal was to manage his symptoms and reduce the side effects of his ongoing treatments.

Over several months, Robert reported fewer side effects and a noticeable improvement in his overall well-being. Blood tests showed stabilized PSA levels, an indicator used to monitor prostate cancer. Robert's case illustrates how complementary approaches can enhance the effectiveness of conventional treatments and improve patient outcomes.

Jessica, a 45-year-old woman with pancreatic cancer, also turned to Dr. Sebi's approach after experiencing limited success with traditional treatments. She embraced the alkaline diet, focusing on organic fruits, vegetables, nuts, and seeds. Jessica also used herbs like chaparral, red clover, and blue vervain, known for their detoxifying and anti-inflammatory properties.

Jessica's condition improved gradually, with scans showing a reduction in tumor size and improved organ function. Her energy levels and appetite increased, and she felt more optimistic about her health journey. Jessica's case further demonstrates the potential of Dr. Sebi's holistic approach to support cancer patients in managing their condition and enhancing their quality of life.

Michael, a 50-year-old man with lung cancer, provides another example of the impact of Dr. Sebi's methods. After facing severe side effects from chemotherapy, Michael decided to adopt the alkaline diet and use herbs such as burdock root, sarsaparilla, and dandelion. He reported a significant reduction in nausea and fatigue, common side effects of his treatment.

Michael's lung function improved, and his overall health stabilized. While he continued with his prescribed medical treatments, the addition of Dr. Sebi's approach provided him with the strength and resilience needed to endure his cancer battle. Michael's case underscores the importance of an integrative approach to cancer care, combining conventional and alternative methods for the best possible outcomes.

These case studies collectively highlight the potential benefits of Dr. Sebi's unconventional approach to cancer treatment. While his methods may not replace conventional treatments, they offer valuable complementary strategies that can improve patient outcomes and quality of life. The emphasis on an alkaline diet and specific herbs provides a holistic framework that supports the body's natural healing processes and enhances overall health.

Dr. Sebi's approach encourages patients to take an active role in their health, focusing on nutrition and natural remedies to complement traditional medical treatments. The positive experiences reported by individuals who have followed his protocol suggest that integrating holistic practices into cancer care can offer hope and improved well-being for many patients. As more people explore these alternative methods, the potential for broader acceptance and integration into mainstream cancer treatment continues to grow.

Treatment for Kidney Stones

Diuretic Herbs and Diet

Treating kidney stones naturally involves using diuretic herbs and a carefully planned diet to facilitate the passage of stones and prevent their formation. Kidney stones, which are hard deposits made of minerals and salts that form inside the kidneys, can cause severe pain and discomfort. A holistic approach to managing kidney stones can provide relief and prevent recurrence by promoting increased urine flow and preventing the crystallization of minerals.

Diuretic herbs play a crucial role in the natural treatment of kidney stones. These herbs help increase urine production, which can aid in flushing out small stones and preventing the formation of new ones. One of the most effective diuretic herbs is dandelion root. Dandelion root is a natural diuretic that helps increase urine output, thereby facilitating the removal of toxins and stones from the kidneys. Consuming dandelion root tea regularly can help maintain healthy kidney function and prevent the buildup of mineral deposits. Another potent diuretic herb is nettle leaf. Nettle leaf not only increases urine production but also helps reduce inflammation in the urinary tract, which can ease the passage of stones. Drinking nettle leaf tea can support overall urinary health and prevent the formation of new stones. Nettle is also rich in essential minerals that support kidney function, making it a valuable addition to a kidney stone prevention regimen.

Parsley is another herb known for its diuretic properties. It helps increase urine flow and can assist in flushing out toxins and small stones from the kidneys. Parsley can be consumed fresh in salads, smoothies, or as a tea. Its mild diuretic effect makes it a safe and effective herb for promoting kidney health.

Horsetail is an ancient herb that has been used for its diuretic properties and ability to support urinary tract health. Horsetail tea can help increase urine output, facilitating the expulsion of small kidney stones. Additionally, horsetail is rich in silica, which supports the health of the urinary tract lining and helps prevent the formation of new stones.

Burdock root is another herb with diuretic and detoxifying properties. It helps cleanse the kidneys and can aid in dissolving small kidney stones. Burdock root tea or supplements can be included in a kidney stone treatment plan to support overall kidney health and prevent recurrence.

Hydration is a fundamental aspect of preventing and treating kidney stones. Drinking plenty of water helps dilute the substances in urine that lead to stones. Aim to drink at least eight to ten glasses of water daily to maintain proper hydration and support kidney function. Adequate water intake can help flush out small stones and prevent the crystallization of minerals that form stones. In addition to using diuretic herbs, dietary changes are crucial for managing kidney stones. Certain foods can either contribute to or prevent the formation of stones, depending on their composition. For instance, foods high in oxalates, such as spinach, beets, and nuts, can contribute to the formation of calcium oxalate stones, the most common type of kidney stone. Limiting the intake of these foods can help reduce the risk of developing new stones.

Conversely, increasing the intake of foods rich in citrate can help prevent stone formation. Citrate binds with calcium in the urine, preventing the formation of calcium crystals. Foods high in citrate include lemons, limes, and other citrus fruits. Drinking lemon water regularly can help increase citrate levels in the urine and reduce the risk of kidney stones.

Calcium intake should not be drastically reduced, as inadequate calcium can lead to increased oxalate absorption and stone formation. Instead, focus on getting calcium from dietary sources rather than supplements. Good dietary sources of calcium include dairy products, leafy greens, and fortified plant-based milk. Pairing calcium-rich foods with meals that contain moderate amounts of oxalates can help reduce the absorption of oxalates.

Magnesium is another important mineral for preventing kidney stones. It helps inhibit the formation of calcium oxalate crystals. Foods rich in magnesium include avocados, bananas, legumes, nuts, and seeds. Ensuring adequate magnesium intake can support overall kidney health and reduce the likelihood of stone formation. A diet low in sodium is also beneficial for preventing kidney stones. High sodium intake can increase calcium levels in the urine, which can contribute to stone formation. Reducing the consumption of processed foods, which are often high in sodium, and avoiding adding extra salt to meals can help maintain lower sodium levels and support kidney health.

Potassium-rich foods can also help prevent kidney stones. Potassium helps regulate fluid balance and supports the proper functioning of the kidneys. Foods high in potassium include bananas, oranges, potatoes, and tomatoes. Including these foods in your diet can help maintain healthy kidney function and reduce the risk of stones.

Protein intake, particularly from animal sources, should be moderated. High protein intake can increase the amount of uric acid in the urine, which can lead to the formation of uric acid stones. Reducing the consumption of red meat, poultry, and seafood, and opting for plant-based protein sources such as legumes, nuts, and seeds can help lower the risk of uric acid stones.

Incorporating more fiber into the diet can also be beneficial for preventing kidney stones. Fiber helps regulate the absorption of calcium and oxalates in the digestive tract. High-fiber foods include fruits, vegetables, whole grains, and legumes. Increasing fiber intake can support digestive health and reduce the risk of stone formation.

In summary, treating kidney stones naturally involves the use of diuretic herbs and dietary modifications to support kidney function and prevent the formation of stones. Herbs such as dandelion root, nettle leaf, parsley, horsetail, and burdock root can help increase urine production and flush out small stones. Adequate hydration, a balanced intake of calcium and magnesium, a diet low in sodium and animal protein, and increased fiber intake are essential strategies for managing kidney stones. By incorporating these natural remedies and dietary changes, individuals can effectively treat and prevent kidney stones, promoting overall kidney health and well-being.

Prevention Strategies

Preventing kidney stones requires a multifaceted approach that combines dietary modifications, lifestyle changes, and the use of specific herbs and supplements. Understanding the factors that contribute to the formation of kidney stones is crucial in developing effective prevention strategies. By addressing these factors, individuals can reduce their risk of developing kidney stones and promote overall kidney health.

Hydration is the cornerstone of kidney stone prevention. Drinking plenty of water dilutes the substances in urine that lead to stones. Aim to drink at least eight to ten glasses of water daily to maintain proper hydration and support kidney function. Adequate hydration helps flush out minerals and prevents them from crystallizing into stones. For those with a history of kidney stones, it may be beneficial to increase water intake further, especially in hot weather or during physical activity. Monitoring urine color can be a simple way to gauge hydration levels. Clear or pale-yellow urine typically indicates good hydration, while darker urine suggests the need for more fluids. Adding lemon or lime to water can increase citrate levels, which helps prevent stone formation. Citrate binds with calcium in the urine, preventing the formation of calcium crystals.

Dietary adjustments are essential for preventing kidney stones. A diet high in oxalates can contribute to the formation of calcium oxalate stones, the most common type of kidney stone. Foods high in oxalates include spinach, beets, nuts, and chocolate. While it's not necessary to eliminate these foods entirely, limiting their intake can help reduce the risk of stone formation. Pairing oxalate-rich foods with calcium-rich foods can help bind oxalates in the digestive tract, reducing their absorption and preventing them from reaching the kidneys.

Calcium intake should come from dietary sources rather than supplements, as excessive calcium supplementation can increase the risk of stones. Good dietary sources of calcium include dairy products, leafy greens, and fortified plant-based milk. Ensuring adequate calcium intake helps prevent the formation of stones by binding with oxalates in the gut and preventing their absorption.

Reducing sodium intake is another important dietary strategy. High sodium levels can increase calcium in the urine, leading to the formation of stones. Reducing sodium intake can help lower calcium levels in the urine. Processed and packaged foods are often high in sodium, so it's essential to read labels and choose low-sodium options. Cooking meals at home and using herbs and spices for flavor instead of salt can also help reduce sodium intake. Limiting animal protein is beneficial for preventing kidney stones, particularly uric acid stones. High protein intake, especially from red meat, poultry, and fish, can increase uric acid levels in the urine, leading to stone formation. Opting for plant-based protein sources like legumes, nuts, and seeds can help lower the risk of uric acid stones. These plant-based proteins are also rich in fiber and other nutrients that support overall health. Increasing the intake of fruits and vegetables is crucial for kidney stone prevention. These foods are high in water content and provide essential vitamins and minerals that support kidney health. They also help maintain an alkaline urine pH, which can prevent the formation of certain types of stones. Citrus fruits, in particular, are beneficial due to their high citrate content, which helps prevent stone formation.

Magnesium is another important mineral for preventing kidney stones. It helps inhibit the formation of calcium oxalate crystals. Foods rich in magnesium include avocados, bananas, legumes, nuts, and seeds. Ensuring adequate magnesium intake can support overall kidney health and reduce the likelihood of stone formation. Magnesium supplements are also available for those who need additional support.

Potassium-rich foods can help prevent kidney stones by supporting proper fluid balance and kidney function. Foods high in potassium include bananas, oranges, potatoes, and tomatoes. Including these foods in your diet can help maintain healthy kidney function and reduce the risk of stones.

Regular physical activity is also important for preventing kidney stones. Exercise helps maintain a healthy weight and supports overall metabolic health, reducing the risk of conditions that can contribute to stone formation. Aim for at least 150 minutes of moderate-intensity exercise per week, such as brisk walking, swimming, or cycling. Strength training exercises are also beneficial as they help build muscle mass and support metabolic health.

Herbal remedies can complement dietary and lifestyle changes in preventing kidney stones. Certain herbs have diuretic properties that increase urine production, helping to flush out small stones and prevent the formation of new ones. Dandelion root, for example, is a natural diuretic that helps increase urine output and maintain healthy kidney function. Drinking dandelion root tea regularly can support kidney health and prevent the buildup of mineral deposits. Nettle leaf is another beneficial herb for kidney stone prevention. It helps increase urine production and reduce inflammation in the urinary tract, making it easier to pass small stones. Drinking nettle leaf tea can support overall urinary health and prevent the formation of new stones. Nettle is also rich in essential minerals that support kidney function. Parsley is known for its mild diuretic effect and can help increase urine flow, aiding in the prevention of kidney stones. Parsley can be consumed fresh in salads, smoothies, or as a tea. Its diuretic properties help flush out toxins and small stones from the kidneys. Horsetail is an ancient herb with diuretic properties that supports urinary tract health. Horsetail tea can help increase urine output, facilitating the expulsion of small kidney stones. Additionally, horsetail is rich in silica, which supports the health of the urinary tract lining and helps prevent the formation of new stones. Burdock root, known for its diuretic and detoxifying properties, can help cleanse the kidneys and dissolve small kidney stones. Burdock root tea or supplements can be included in a kidney stone prevention plan to support overall kidney health and prevent recurrence.

Monitoring and adjusting dietary oxalate, calcium, sodium, and protein intake, staying hydrated, incorporating regular exercise, and using specific herbs are comprehensive strategies to prevent kidney stones. This holistic approach not only supports kidney health but also promotes overall well-being. By making these lifestyle and dietary changes, individuals can effectively reduce their risk of developing kidney stones and enhance their quality of life.

Treatment for Other Diseases

Autoimmune Diseases

Autoimmune diseases occur when the body's immune system mistakenly attacks its own tissues, leading to chronic inflammation and a host of debilitating symptoms. Conditions such as rheumatoid arthritis, lupus, multiple sclerosis, and Hashimoto's thyroiditis fall under this category. Treatment of autoimmune diseases requires a holistic approach that aims to reduce inflammation, balance the immune system, and support overall health. Diet, lifestyle modifications, and herbal remedies play crucial roles in managing these conditions effectively.

A primary strategy in treating autoimmune diseases is to adopt an anti-inflammatory diet. This type of diet focuses on consuming foods that reduce inflammation and avoiding those that can trigger it. Fresh fruits and vegetables are key components because they are rich in antioxidants and phytonutrients that help combat oxidative stress and inflammation. Leafy greens, berries, and cruciferous vegetables like broccoli and cauliflower are particularly beneficial. Healthy fats, such as those found in avocados, nuts, seeds, and olive oil, also play an essential role in reducing inflammation. Omega-3 fatty acids, present in fatty fish like salmon and mackerel, as well as in flaxseeds and chia seeds, have powerful anti-inflammatory properties. Including these fats in the diet can help modulate the immune response and reduce the severity of autoimmune symptoms.

Protein is another crucial element, but it's important to choose the right sources. Lean proteins like poultry, fish, and plant-based proteins such as legumes and tofu are excellent choices. These proteins support muscle repair and immune function without contributing to inflammation. In contrast, it's important to avoid foods that can exacerbate inflammation. Processed foods, refined sugars, trans fats, and excessive alcohol consumption can all trigger inflammatory responses in the body. Gluten and dairy are also common culprits that can provoke autoimmune flare-ups in some individuals. Eliminating or significantly reducing these foods from the diet can help alleviate symptoms and improve overall health. In addition to dietary changes, certain herbs have been shown to be beneficial in managing autoimmune diseases. Turmeric, with its active compound curcumin, is one of the most potent anti-inflammatory herbs. Curcumin can help reduce joint pain and swelling in conditions like rheumatoid arthritis. Incorporating turmeric into the diet, either through cooking or supplements, can provide significant relief.

Ginger is another herb with strong anti-inflammatory properties. It can help reduce pain and inflammation in autoimmune conditions. Fresh ginger can be added to teas, smoothies, and meals, or taken as a supplement to harness its benefits.

Ashwagandha, an adaptogenic herb, is known for its ability to balance the immune system and reduce stress. It can help manage autoimmune symptoms by modulating the immune response and reducing cortisol levels. Ashwagandha can be taken in supplement form or as a tea to support overall health.

Aloe vera is beneficial for autoimmune conditions that affect the skin, such as psoriasis and lupus. Aloe vera gel can be applied topically to soothe inflammation and promote healing. Additionally, aloe vera juice can be consumed to support digestive health and reduce internal inflammation.

Stress management is another critical component in treating autoimmune diseases. Chronic stress can exacerbate symptoms and trigger flare-ups. Practices such as meditation, yoga, and deep breathing exercises can help reduce stress and improve mental well-being. Regular physical activity is also beneficial, as it helps reduce inflammation, boost mood, and improve overall health. Getting adequate sleep is essential for managing autoimmune diseases. Poor sleep can worsen symptoms and weaken the immune system. Aim for seven to nine hours of quality sleep each night and establish a consistent sleep routine. Creating a relaxing bedtime environment and avoiding stimulants like caffeine before bed can help improve sleep quality.

Detoxification can also support the management of autoimmune diseases. The accumulation of toxins in the body can trigger inflammatory responses and worsen symptoms. Regular detox practices, such as drinking plenty of water, consuming detoxifying herbs like dandelion and milk thistle, and engaging in activities that promote sweating, like saunas or exercise, can help eliminate toxins and support overall health. In addition to these strategies, it is important to work closely with healthcare providers to develop a comprehensive treatment plan tailored to individual needs. Regular monitoring of symptoms, adjusting treatments as necessary, and staying informed about new developments in autoimmune disease management can help individuals maintain a better quality of life.

Overall, treating autoimmune diseases involves a multifaceted approach that includes dietary changes, herbal remedies, stress management, sleep optimization, and detoxification. By adopting these strategies, individuals can reduce inflammation, balance their immune system, and improve their overall health and well-being. This holistic approach offers a natural and effective way to manage autoimmune diseases and enhance quality of life.

Digestive Disorders

Digestive disorders encompass a wide range of conditions affecting the gastrointestinal tract, including irritable bowel syndrome (IBS), Crohn's disease, ulcerative colitis, and gastroesophageal reflux disease (GERD). These conditions can significantly impact a person's quality of life, causing symptoms such as abdominal pain, bloating, diarrhea, constipation, and heartburn. Managing digestive disorders requires a comprehensive approach that includes dietary changes, lifestyle modifications, and the use of natural remedies to support digestive health and alleviate symptoms.

One of the most effective strategies for managing digestive disorders is adopting a diet that supports gut health. This involves consuming foods that are easy to digest and nourish the gut microbiome, the community of beneficial bacteria in the intestines. Fermented foods such as yogurt, kefir, sauerkraut, kimchi, and kombucha are rich in probiotics, which help maintain a healthy balance of gut bacteria. These beneficial bacteria aid in digestion, enhance nutrient absorption, and protect against harmful pathogens. In addition to fermented foods, incorporating prebiotic-rich foods into the diet is essential. Prebiotics are non-digestible fibers that serve as food for probiotics, promoting their growth and activity. Foods high in prebiotics include garlic, onions, leeks, asparagus, bananas, and whole grains. Including these foods in the diet can help improve gut health and alleviate symptoms of digestive disorders.

Fiber is another crucial component of a digestive-friendly diet. Soluble fiber, found in foods like oats, legumes, apples, and carrots, absorbs water and forms a gel-like substance in the intestines, which helps regulate bowel movements and prevent constipation. Insoluble fiber, found in whole grains, nuts, seeds, and vegetables, adds bulk to the stool and promotes regularity. A balanced intake of both types of fiber can help manage symptoms of IBS, constipation, and other digestive disorders.

Hydration is also vital for digestive health. Drinking plenty of water helps maintain the consistency of stool and prevents dehydration, which can exacerbate digestive issues. Herbal teas, such as peppermint, ginger, and chamomile, can provide additional digestive benefits. Peppermint tea has antispasmodic properties that can help relieve symptoms of IBS, while ginger tea can reduce nausea and improve digestion. Chamomile tea has anti-inflammatory and calming effects that can soothe the digestive tract and reduce symptoms of GERD. Eliminating or reducing foods that can trigger digestive symptoms is also important. Common trigger foods include high-fat and fried foods, spicy foods, caffeine, alcohol, and artificial sweeteners. Keeping a food diary can help identify specific triggers and guide dietary adjustments to minimize symptoms. For individuals with lactose intolerance, avoiding dairy products or choosing lactose-free alternatives can prevent symptoms such as bloating, gas, and diarrhea. In addition to dietary changes, certain natural remedies can help manage digestive disorders. One such remedy is aloe vera juice, which has soothing and anti-inflammatory properties that can help heal the lining of the digestive tract and reduce symptoms of GERD and IBS. Aloe vera juice should be consumed in moderation, as excessive intake can have a laxative effect.

Slippery elm is another herbal remedy known for its soothing effects on the digestive system. It contains mucilage, a gel-like substance that coats and protects the lining of the intestines, reducing inflammation and irritation. Slippery elm can be taken as a tea or in supplement form to alleviate symptoms of IBS, Crohn's disease, and ulcerative colitis.

Licorice root, specifically deglycyrrhizinated licorice (DGL), is beneficial for digestive health. DGL can help reduce inflammation and promote the healing of the stomach lining, making it useful for managing GERD and peptic ulcers. It can be taken in chewable tablet form before meals to provide relief from heartburn and indigestion.

For individuals with IBS, peppermint oil capsules can be an effective remedy. Peppermint oil has antispasmodic properties that can relax the muscles of the intestines and reduce symptoms such as abdominal pain, bloating, and gas. Enteric-coated peppermint oil capsules are designed to dissolve in the intestines rather than the stomach, minimizing the risk of heartburn.

Stress management is another crucial aspect of managing digestive disorders. Stress can exacerbate symptoms and disrupt normal digestive function. Practices such as mindfulness meditation, deep breathing exercises, yoga, and tai chi can help reduce stress and promote relaxation. Regular physical activity is also beneficial for digestive health, as it helps stimulate bowel movements and reduce symptoms of constipation.

Adequate sleep is essential for maintaining overall health, including digestive health. Poor sleep can worsen symptoms of digestive disorders and contribute to stress and anxiety. Establishing a regular sleep routine, creating a relaxing bedtime environment, and avoiding stimulants like caffeine before bed can help improve sleep quality.

In summary, managing digestive disorders involves a multifaceted approach that includes dietary changes, natural remedies, and lifestyle modifications. Consuming a diet rich in fiber, probiotics, and prebiotics, staying hydrated, and avoiding trigger foods can support gut health and alleviate symptoms. Natural remedies such as aloe vera juice, slippery elm, licorice root, and peppermint oil can provide additional relief. Stress management, regular physical activity, and adequate sleep are also crucial for maintaining digestive health. By adopting these strategies, individuals with digestive disorders can improve their symptoms and enhance their overall quality of life. This holistic approach offers a natural and effective way to manage digestive disorders and promote long-term gut health.

Skin Problems

Skin problems can range from minor irritations to chronic conditions that significantly impact an individual's quality of life. Conditions such as eczema, psoriasis, acne, and rosacea can be particularly distressing. Effective treatment of these skin issues involves a combination of dietary changes, natural topical treatments, and lifestyle modifications to promote skin health and address underlying causes.

Diet plays a crucial role in maintaining healthy skin. Consuming a diet rich in vitamins, minerals, and antioxidants can help improve skin condition and reduce the symptoms of various skin problems. Fresh fruits and vegetables are essential for providing these nutrients. Foods high in vitamins A, C, and E, such as carrots, sweet potatoes, citrus fruits, and leafy greens, support skin health by promoting collagen production, protecting against UV damage, and reducing inflammation.

Omega-3 fatty acids are another critical component of a skin-healthy diet. Found in fatty fish like salmon and mackerel, as well as in flaxseeds and walnuts, omega-3s help reduce inflammation and keep the skin moisturized. Including these foods in your diet can help alleviate symptoms of eczema and psoriasis, which are often exacerbated by inflammation and dryness.

Hydration is also fundamental for healthy skin. Drinking plenty of water helps maintain skin's elasticity and suppleness. It supports the skin's barrier function, preventing dryness and irritation. Herbal teas, particularly those with anti-inflammatory properties like chamomile and green tea, can also contribute to skin hydration and health.

Topical treatments using natural ingredients can provide significant relief for various skin problems. Aloe vera is a versatile remedy known for its soothing and healing properties. It can be applied directly to the skin to reduce inflammation, moisturize, and promote healing. Aloe vera is particularly effective for conditions like eczema and psoriasis, where inflammation and dryness are primary concerns.

Honey is another powerful natural remedy for skin problems. It has antibacterial and anti-inflammatory properties, making it effective for treating acne and soothing irritated skin. Raw honey can be applied as a mask to help clear up acne, reduce redness, and promote a healthy complexion.

Coconut oil is a popular treatment for dry skin conditions such as eczema. It has moisturizing and antimicrobial properties that help soothe and protect the skin. Applying coconut oil to affected areas can provide relief from itching and prevent infections caused by scratching.

Tea tree oil is well-known for its antiseptic and anti-inflammatory properties. It is particularly useful for treating acne due to its ability to kill acne-causing bacteria and reduce inflammation. Diluting tea tree oil with a carrier oil, such as jojoba or almond oil, and applying it to blemishes can help clear up acne and prevent future breakouts.

Oatmeal is another natural ingredient that can be used to treat skin problems. Colloidal oatmeal, which is finely ground oatmeal, can be added to baths or used in creams and lotions to soothe irritated skin and reduce inflammation. It is especially beneficial for conditions like eczema and dermatitis.

Dietary changes and topical treatments are often complemented by lifestyle modifications to achieve the best results in managing skin problems. Stress management is crucial, as stress can trigger or exacerbate conditions like acne, eczema, and psoriasis. Techniques such as yoga, meditation, and deep breathing exercises can help reduce stress and improve overall skin health.

Adequate sleep is essential for skin regeneration and repair. Poor sleep can lead to increased stress levels and exacerbate skin problems. Aim for seven to nine hours of quality sleep each night to support skin health. Creating a consistent sleep routine and a relaxing bedtime environment can help improve sleep quality.

Exercise is another important factor in maintaining healthy skin. Regular physical activity promotes circulation, which helps deliver oxygen and nutrients to the skin. Exercise also helps reduce stress and improve overall health, contributing to better skin condition. Aim for at least 30 minutes of moderate exercise most days of the week.

Protecting the skin from environmental damage is also important in managing skin problems. Using natural sunscreens to protect against UV damage, wearing protective clothing, and avoiding excessive exposure to harsh weather conditions can help prevent flare-ups and maintain healthy skin.

In addition to these strategies, certain herbs can be used both internally and externally to support skin health. Burdock root, for example, is known for its detoxifying properties and can be taken as a tea or supplement to help cleanse the blood and improve skin condition. Topically, burdock root can be used in salves and creams to reduce inflammation and promote healing.

Calendula, also known as marigold, is a herb with powerful anti-inflammatory and healing properties. Calendula oil or cream can be applied to the skin to soothe irritation, reduce inflammation, and promote healing. It is particularly effective for conditions like eczema, dermatitis, and minor wounds.

Turmeric, with its active compound curcumin, is another beneficial herb for skin health. Turmeric can be taken internally as a supplement or added to food to reduce inflammation and support overall health. Topically, turmeric paste can be applied to the skin to reduce inflammation and promote healing.

Gotu kola is a herb traditionally used in Ayurvedic medicine for its skin-healing properties. It can be taken as a supplement or applied topically in creams and lotions to improve skin elasticity, promote healing, and reduce the appearance of scars and stretch marks.

Integrating these dietary changes, natural topical treatments, lifestyle modifications, and herbal remedies can provide a comprehensive approach to managing skin problems. By addressing both the symptoms and underlying causes of skin conditions, individuals can achieve healthier, clearer skin and improve their overall quality of life. This holistic approach not only treats the skin externally but also promotes internal health, leading to long-term benefits for skin health and overall well-being.

Part 6: Testimonials and Case Studies

Success Stories

Testimonials from people who followed Dr. Sebi's protocols

The transformative power of Dr. Sebi's protocols has touched countless lives, reshaping health narratives in ways conventional medicine often struggles to comprehend. The stories of those who have embraced his alkaline diet and herbal remedies offer profound insights into the potential for natural healing. These success stories serve not just as testimonials but as living proof of the efficacy of holistic health approaches, inspiring others to embark on their journeys toward wellness.

One such story is that of Maria Lopez, a 45-year-old woman from Los Angeles who had been battling severe arthritis for over a decade. Her condition had progressively worsened despite various medical treatments, leaving her in constant pain and with limited mobility. Frustrated and desperate for relief, Maria stumbled upon Dr. Sebi's teachings online. Skeptical yet hopeful, she decided to give the alkaline diet a try. Within a few weeks, she noticed a remarkable reduction in inflammation and pain. Her joints became more flexible, and she could perform daily tasks that had once seemed impossible. Maria's story is not just about alleviating symptoms; it's about reclaiming a quality of life she thought she had lost forever.

Similarly, Robert Mitchell, a 32-year-old tech professional, found himself grappling with chronic fatigue and digestive issues. Despite being active and seemingly healthy, he often felt drained and struggled with stomach discomfort that interfered with his work and personal life. Conventional doctors attributed his symptoms to stress and prescribed medications that offered little relief. It was only after a friend recommended Dr. Sebi's approach that Robert saw a glimmer of hope. Transitioning to an alkaline diet and incorporating specific herbs into his routine, Robert experienced a significant boost in energy levels and a marked improvement in his digestive health. He felt revitalized, more focused, and capable of performing at his best, both professionally and personally.

Then there's the compelling case of Samantha Greene, a 27-year-old diagnosed with polycystic ovary syndrome (PCOS). For years, Samantha dealt with irregular menstrual cycles, severe acne, and weight gain, conditions that conventional treatments seemed to only partially address. After extensive research, she found Dr. Sebi's philosophy intriguing and decided to adopt his dietary guidelines and herbal treatments. Within six months, Samantha's menstrual cycles became regular, her skin cleared up, and she lost the excess weight that had plagued her. Her story underscores the potential for natural remedies to restore hormonal balance and overall well-being.

Equally inspiring is the journey of Harold Thompson, a retired teacher who had been diagnosed with type 2 diabetes. Managing his blood sugar levels had become a daily struggle, and the side effects of his medications were taking a toll on his health. Upon learning about Dr. Sebi's success in treating diabetes through diet and herbs, Harold was determined to follow this alternative path. Gradually, he replaced processed foods with nutrient-rich, alkaline options and incorporated herbal supplements into his regimen. The results were astonishing. Harold's blood sugar levels stabilized, and he was able to reduce, and eventually eliminate, his reliance on insulin. His energy and vitality returned, allowing him to enjoy his retirement fully and pursue his passions without the constant burden of managing his condition.

Another poignant account is that of Lisa Morgan, a young mother who faced the harrowing challenge of her son's eczema. Her son, Ethan, had severe eczema that caused him immense discomfort and affected his sleep and daily activities. Traditional treatments provided only temporary relief, and Lisa was determined to find a lasting solution. Upon discovering Dr. Sebi's emphasis on the relationship between diet and skin health, she overhauled Ethan's diet and incorporated recommended herbs. The change was nothing short of miraculous. Ethan's eczema began to heal, his skin cleared up, and he could sleep through the night without itching. Lisa's relief and joy were immeasurable, and she became a fervent advocate for holistic health, sharing her son's success story with other parents facing similar challenges.

The narrative of John Matthews, a 60-year-old former athlete suffering from debilitating heart disease, further illustrates the potential of Dr. Sebi's protocols. Years of rigorous training had taken a toll on his heart, and conventional treatments offered limited hope. John was introduced to Dr. Sebi's philosophy by a fellow athlete and decided to adopt an alkaline diet combined with specific heart-strengthening herbs. Over time, his cholesterol levels improved, blood pressure normalized, and overall cardiovascular health showed significant enhancement. John felt rejuvenated, able to engage in physical activities he had long abandoned and living proof that even chronic conditions could be managed through natural means.

These success stories highlight the profound impact of Dr. Sebi's approach on various health conditions, but they also emphasize a deeper, more personal transformation. The individuals who have embraced these protocols often describe a renewed sense of empowerment and control over their health. They speak of a holistic awakening, where the mind, body, and spirit are harmonized through natural means. The stories are not just about physical healing; they are about the resurgence of hope, vitality, and a redefined relationship with food and nature.

The journey of adopting Dr. Sebi's protocols is rarely easy. It requires a significant shift in mindset, lifestyle, and daily habits. Many of those who have succeeded credit their perseverance and the support of a community that shares similar beliefs. They often highlight the importance of education and awareness, advocating for others to explore these natural alternatives as viable options for health and wellness.

The success stories of individuals like Maria, Robert, Samantha, Harold, Lisa, and John serve as powerful testaments to the potential of natural healing. They offer a glimpse into the transformative power of an alkaline diet and herbal remedies, inspiring others to explore these methods and embark on their healing journeys. Through these narratives, the legacy of Dr. Sebi continues to thrive, touching lives and fostering a deeper understanding of holistic health.

Detailed Case Studies

In delving deeper into the life-altering journeys of those who have adhered to Dr. Sebi's protocols, we uncover profound narratives that highlight not only individual triumphs over chronic illnesses but also the intricate process of transformation. These detailed case studies provide an intimate look at the perseverance, challenges, and ultimate success experienced by people who embraced natural healing methods.

Consider the case of Charles Bennett, a 52-year-old businessman from Atlanta who had been diagnosed with high blood pressure and high cholesterol. Despite adhering to a conventional medical regimen prescribed by his doctors, Charles found himself trapped in a cycle of dependency on medications, which seemed to provide little more than temporary relief. Frustrated by the side effects and lack of sustainable improvement, Charles began exploring alternative therapies. His research led him to Dr. Sebi's philosophy, and he was particularly drawn to the concept of restoring the body's natural pH balance through diet.

Charles began his journey by meticulously researching the alkaline diet and Dr. Sebi's recommended herbs. He transitioned gradually, eliminating processed foods and incorporating nutrient-dense, alkaline-rich vegetables, fruits, and herbs into his meals. The initial phase was challenging, as he had to navigate through a complete overhaul of his eating habits. However, within a few months, Charles started noticing significant changes. His blood pressure levels began to stabilize, and he experienced a noticeable decrease in cholesterol levels. More importantly, he felt a renewed sense of energy and mental clarity that he hadn't experienced in years. The success of Charles' case was not merely in the numbers but in the qualitative improvement of his daily life.

Equally compelling is the story of Margaret Hill, a 38-year-old mother of two who had struggled with severe migraines since her teenage years. These debilitating headaches had affected her ability to work, care for her children, and maintain a social life. Traditional medications provided temporary relief but did not address the underlying causes, leaving Margaret in a perpetual state of frustration and pain. A chance conversation with a colleague introduced her to Dr. Sebi's teachings. Intrigued, Margaret decided to dive deeper into the potential of natural remedies.

Margaret's approach was holistic. She adopted the alkaline diet with a particular focus on hydration and the elimination of trigger foods identified in Dr. Sebi's guidelines. She also incorporated specific herbs known for their anti-inflammatory and detoxifying properties. The transition wasn't easy, especially with the demands of motherhood, but Margaret remained committed. Over time, the frequency and intensity of her migraines began to diminish. The turning point came when she realized she had gone an entire month without a single migraine—a feat she hadn't achieved in over two decades. Margaret's story underscores the potential of natural interventions to bring about profound relief where conventional medicine often falls short.

Another illustrative case is that of Jonathan Reed, a young athlete who developed chronic bronchitis following a severe respiratory infection. Jonathan's condition severely impacted his athletic performance and overall quality of life. Despite numerous courses of antibiotics and other medications, his symptoms persisted. Desperate for a solution, Jonathan's coach recommended exploring Dr. Sebi's approach, particularly the emphasis on mucus reduction and lung health.

Jonathan embraced the alkaline diet and started using herbs such as mullein and eucalyptus, known for their respiratory benefits. He also engaged in regular breathing exercises and detoxification practices recommended by Dr. Sebi. The journey was arduous, marked by periods of doubt and difficulty. However, Jonathan's persistence paid off. Gradually, his symptoms began to improve. His breathing became easier, and he was able to resume his training with renewed vigor. Jonathan's recovery wasn't just about returning to sports; it was about reclaiming his health and the passion that defined his life.

The case of Ellen Foster, a 55-year-old librarian from Chicago, further exemplifies the transformative power of Dr. Sebi's protocols. Ellen had been battling with severe depression and anxiety for most of her adult life. Traditional therapies, including medications and counseling, offered limited relief, and she found herself in a constant struggle with her mental health. Ellen discovered Dr. Sebi's work through a support group focused on natural healing methods. Skeptical but hopeful, she decided to give it a try.

Ellen's journey involved a comprehensive approach. She adopted the alkaline diet, focusing on foods that promoted mental clarity and emotional well-being.

Additionally, she incorporated herbs known for their calming and mood-stabilizing effects, such as chamomile and valerian root. Ellen also embraced mindfulness practices and regular physical activity. The transformation was gradual but profound. Over the course of a year, Ellen's depressive episodes became less frequent and severe. She found herself more resilient in the face of stress and more engaged with her work and social life. Ellen's story is a testament to the potential for natural approaches to provide holistic mental health support.

These detailed case studies are not just isolated success stories; they illustrate a broader narrative about the potential of natural healing methods. The common thread in each of these journeys is the commitment to a holistic approach that goes beyond symptom management to address underlying imbalances and promote overall wellness. The individuals who embraced Dr. Sebi's protocols often had to navigate significant lifestyle changes, but the rewards were well worth the effort.

In exploring these narratives, we see a recurring theme of empowerment. Those who followed Dr. Sebi's teachings did more than just adopt a diet; they embraced a philosophy of health that emphasized the body's innate ability to heal when provided with the right conditions. Their journeys were marked by perseverance, education, and a willingness to explore alternatives beyond conventional medicine.

These case studies offer valuable insights for anyone considering natural healing methods. They highlight the importance of patience, consistency, and a holistic approach to health. The successes of Charles, Margaret, Jonathan, and Ellen are not just about overcoming specific conditions; they are about transforming lives through the power of natural healing. Their stories inspire and provide a roadmap for others seeking to reclaim their health and well-being through holistic practices.

Part 7: Additional Resources

FAQ

Answers to Common Questions about Dr. Sebi's Diet and Practices

Navigating the landscape of Dr. Sebi's diet and practices often raises numerous questions, especially for those new to the concept of an alkaline lifestyle. The principles behind this holistic approach can be both intriguing and perplexing, leading to a multitude of inquiries about its efficacy, safety, and practicality. Here, we address some of the most frequently asked questions, providing clarity and insight into Dr. Sebi's unique philosophy.

One of the most common questions is, "What exactly is the alkaline diet, and how does it differ from other diets?" The alkaline diet, as advocated by Dr. Sebi, focuses on consuming foods that maintain a balanced pH level in the body. This involves eating primarily plant-based, alkaline-forming foods and avoiding acid-forming foods. The key difference between this diet and others is its emphasis on the body's internal pH balance. While many diets focus on calorie counting or macronutrient ratios, the alkaline diet prioritizes the consumption of natural, unprocessed foods that promote an alkaline state, which is believed to prevent disease and enhance overall health.

Another frequent question revolves around the types of foods that are allowed and those that should be avoided. People often wonder, "Can I eat fruits and vegetables on the alkaline diet?" The answer is a resounding yes, but with specific guidelines. Not all fruits and vegetables are considered equal in the context of the alkaline diet. Dr. Sebi's approved food list includes alkaline-forming items such as berries, melons, leafy greens, and certain root vegetables. Conversely, acidic foods like tomatoes, oranges, and certain grains are discouraged. This selective approach aims to optimize the body's pH levels and reduce acidity, which is linked to various health issues.

A related question is, "Why are certain healthy foods like tomatoes and oranges excluded from the diet?" The exclusion of these foods often confuses those who have long considered them healthy staples. Dr. Sebi's rationale is based on their acid-forming properties. While these foods are nutritious and beneficial in many diets, within the framework of the alkaline diet, they are believed to contribute to an acidic environment in the body, potentially leading to inflammation and other health problems. Therefore, the focus is on consuming foods that are inherently alkaline to maintain the desired pH balance.

Many individuals are curious about the potential benefits they can expect from following Dr. Sebi's diet. A common inquiry is, "What health improvements can I anticipate?" Followers of the alkaline diet report a wide range of health benefits, from increased energy levels and improved digestion to enhanced mental clarity and better skin health. Additionally, many have experienced relief from chronic conditions such as hypertension, diabetes, and arthritis. The diet's emphasis on whole, nutrient-dense foods helps reduce inflammation and supports the body's natural detoxification processes, leading to these positive outcomes.

Safety is another major concern for those considering a significant dietary shift. People often ask, "Is the alkaline diet safe for everyone?" Generally, the diet is safe for most individuals, as it promotes the consumption of whole, unprocessed foods that are beneficial for overall health. However, it is essential to approach any major dietary change with caution and, ideally, under the guidance of a healthcare professional, especially for individuals with preexisting medical conditions or those who are pregnant or breastfeeding. Customizing the diet to meet individual needs and ensuring a balanced intake of essential nutrients are crucial for maintaining health and well-being.

Practicality and accessibility of the diet are also frequent topics of concern. Many people wonder, "Is it difficult to find and prepare alkaline foods?" While it may seem daunting at first, with some planning and effort, following the alkaline diet can become a seamless part of daily life. Farmers' markets, health food stores, and online retailers often carry the recommended foods and herbs. Learning to prepare meals using these ingredients can be a rewarding experience, fostering a deeper connection with the food and its health benefits. Numerous recipes and resources are available to help individuals incorporate these foods into their diet creatively and deliciously.

A recurring question among newcomers is, "How soon can I expect to see results?" The timeline for experiencing benefits from the alkaline diet varies from person to person, depending on their initial health status and adherence to the dietary guidelines. Some individuals report noticeable improvements within a few weeks, while others may take several months to experience significant changes. Patience and consistency are key, as the body gradually adjusts to the new dietary regimen and begins to heal and detoxify.

People also ask about the scientific backing of Dr. Sebi's principles, with questions like, "Is there scientific evidence supporting the alkaline diet?" While there is ongoing debate within the medical community about the impact of diet on body pH, numerous studies highlight the benefits of a plant-based diet rich in fruits, vegetables, and whole grains. These foods are known to reduce inflammation, improve metabolic health, and lower the risk of chronic diseases. However, it is important to note that the specific claims of the alkaline diet, particularly regarding its ability to cure diseases, are not universally accepted and require further scientific investigation.

Another important question is, "Can I still enjoy social activities and dining out while following the alkaline diet?" Social situations and eating out can pose challenges, but they are not insurmountable. Many restaurants offer plant-based options or are willing to accommodate dietary requests. Planning ahead, such as reviewing menus online or suggesting restaurants with healthy options, can make dining out more manageable. Additionally, educating friends and family about your dietary choices can foster understanding and support, making social interactions more enjoyable and less stressful.

Lastly, people often seek guidance on staying motivated and committed to the diet. They ask, "How can I maintain consistency with the alkaline diet?" Staying committed requires a strong personal motivation and understanding of the diet's benefits. Keeping a food journal, setting realistic goals, and celebrating small victories can help maintain momentum. Joining online communities or local support groups can provide additional encouragement and resources, creating a network of like-minded individuals who share similar health goals.

In addressing these common questions, it becomes evident that Dr. Sebi's diet and practices offer a unique approach to health and wellness. The emphasis on natural, alkaline-forming foods and herbs provides a foundation for improving overall well-being. By understanding the principles behind this holistic approach and addressing concerns with practical solutions, individuals can navigate their journey toward better health with confidence and clarity.

Debunking Common Myths

When it comes to Dr. Sebi's diet and practices, there are numerous misconceptions that can create confusion and skepticism. Addressing these myths with clear, evidence-based explanations is essential for understanding the true potential of this holistic approach to health.

One pervasive myth is that the alkaline diet is merely a trend with no scientific backing. This notion stems from the diet's emphasis on the body's pH balance, which some critics argue is not significantly influenced by food. However, while it's true that the body's blood pH is tightly regulated, the foods we consume can affect the pH of our urine and saliva, which reflects our body's overall state. The alkaline diet promotes the consumption of natural, plant-based foods that are known to reduce inflammation and support overall health. These dietary choices can lead to improved metabolic functions and a reduced risk of chronic diseases, lending credence to the principles behind the alkaline diet.

Another common myth is that Dr. Sebi's diet lacks sufficient protein and other essential nutrients, making it nutritionally inadequate. This misconception often arises from the diet's exclusion of animal products and certain common foods. However, the diet encourages the consumption of a wide variety of plant-based foods rich in protein, such as quinoa, hemp seeds, and leafy greens. Additionally, many of the approved foods are high in essential vitamins, minerals, and antioxidants. By diversifying their intake of these nutrient-dense foods, individuals can meet their nutritional needs while adhering to the diet's guidelines.

There is also a belief that Dr. Sebi's diet is too restrictive and difficult to follow. This perception is understandable, given the specific list of approved and forbidden foods. However, many followers find that the diet becomes easier to manage with time and practice. By focusing on the wide array of allowed foods, such as fruits, vegetables, nuts, seeds, and grains, individuals can create diverse and satisfying meals. Learning to prepare these foods in creative ways can make the diet enjoyable and sustainable. Furthermore, the health benefits experienced by many adherents often provide strong motivation to continue.

Some people argue that Dr. Sebi's diet is expensive and not accessible to everyone. While it is true that organic and wildcrafted foods can be more costly than conventional options, there are ways to make the diet more affordable. Buying in bulk, shopping at farmers' markets, and growing one's own herbs and vegetables can help reduce costs. Additionally, the investment in high-quality, nutrient-dense foods can lead to long-term savings on healthcare expenses by preventing chronic diseases and reducing the need for medications.

A prevalent myth is that Dr. Sebi's approach lacks scientific validation and relies solely on anecdotal evidence. While more research is needed to fully understand the mechanisms behind the alkaline diet, numerous studies support the health benefits of a plant-based diet rich in fruits, vegetables, and whole grains. These foods have been shown to lower the risk of chronic diseases, improve digestive health, and support the body's natural detoxification processes. Moreover, many followers of Dr. Sebi's diet report significant improvements in their health, providing a strong body of anecdotal evidence that complements existing scientific research.

Another myth is that herbs recommended by Dr. Sebi are not effective and can be harmful. This misconception often arises from a lack of understanding about the properties and uses of these herbs. Many of the herbs recommended by Dr. Sebi, such as burdock root, sarsaparilla, and bladderwrack, have been used traditionally for their medicinal properties and are supported by scientific research. These herbs are known for their anti-inflammatory, detoxifying, and immune-boosting effects. When used properly, they can complement the alkaline diet and support overall health. However, it is important to use herbs with caution and under the guidance of a knowledgeable healthcare provider.

Some skeptics claim that Dr. Sebi's diet and practices are a form of pseudoscience and that following them is akin to rejecting conventional medicine. This binary thinking fails to recognize the value of integrating natural and conventional approaches to health. Dr. Sebi's diet promotes the use of whole, unprocessed foods and natural remedies to support the body's healing processes, which can complement conventional treatments. Many individuals find that incorporating these holistic practices enhances their overall health and well-being, allowing them to reduce their reliance on medications and improve their quality of life.

A frequently encountered myth is that the benefits of Dr. Sebi's diet are purely placebo effects. While the placebo effect can play a role in any health intervention, the tangible improvements reported by many followers of the diet suggest that there is more at play. The diet's emphasis on nutrient-dense, anti-inflammatory foods and detoxifying herbs can have profound physiological effects, supporting the body's natural healing processes. The consistent health improvements observed by adherents, including increased energy levels, weight loss, and reduced symptoms of chronic conditions, indicate that the diet's benefits are real and substantial.

Lastly, there is a misconception that the alkaline diet is only suitable for those with specific health conditions and not for the general population. While the diet has gained attention for its potential to address chronic illnesses, its principles can benefit anyone seeking to improve their overall health. The focus on whole, plant-based foods and natural remedies can enhance metabolic function, boost the immune system, and promote longevity. By adopting the diet's guidelines, individuals from all walks of life can experience improved vitality and well-being.

In debunking these common myths, it becomes clear that Dr. Sebi's diet and practices offer a viable approach to health that is grounded in both tradition and emerging scientific understanding. The emphasis on natural, nutrient-dense foods and herbal remedies provides a framework for achieving and maintaining optimal health. By addressing misconceptions and providing accurate information, we can help more people explore and benefit from this holistic approach to wellness.

Useful Resources

List of Herb Suppliers

Embarking on a journey with Dr. Sebi's alkaline diet and herbal practices requires not just dedication but also access to high-quality resources. One of the most critical components is sourcing the herbs that are central to many of Dr. Sebi's protocols. Finding reliable herb suppliers can significantly influence the effectiveness of the treatments and overall health benefits. The following guide highlights some of the most reputable sources for these essential herbs, ensuring you receive products that are both authentic and potent.

Starting your search for herbs, it's crucial to understand the different types of suppliers available. There are various avenues you can explore, from local herb shops to online retailers, each offering unique advantages. Local herb shops provide the benefit of in-person consultations and the ability to inspect products before purchasing. These shops often employ knowledgeable staff who can offer personalized advice and recommendations based on your specific needs. Visiting a local herb shop can also foster a sense of community and support as you connect with others who share your interest in natural healing.

On the other hand, online retailers offer unparalleled convenience and a wider selection of herbs. When choosing an online supplier, it is essential to prioritize those with a reputation for quality and transparency. Look for companies that provide detailed information about the sourcing, harvesting, and processing of their herbs. Many reputable online suppliers also offer third-party lab testing results, ensuring their products are free from contaminants and meet high standards of purity and potency. This level of transparency not only builds trust but also assures you of the product's efficacy.

One of the well-regarded online suppliers is Mountain Rose Herbs. Known for their commitment to organic and sustainably sourced products, Mountain Rose Herbs offers an extensive range of herbs, including many recommended by Dr. Sebi. Their website provides comprehensive information about each herb, including its uses, benefits, and recommended preparations. Additionally, they offer various forms of herbs, such as dried, powdered, and liquid extracts, catering to different preferences and needs.

Another excellent resource is Starwest Botanicals. With a history dating back to 1975, Starwest Botanicals has built a solid reputation for quality and integrity. They offer a broad selection of herbs, spices, and essential oils, many of which are organic and wildcrafted. Their commitment to quality is evident in their rigorous testing procedures and certifications, ensuring that customers receive only the best products. Starwest Botanicals also provides educational resources, helping customers make informed choices about the herbs they purchase.

For those looking for wildcrafted herbs, Pacific Botanicals is a noteworthy supplier. Specializing in organically grown and wildcrafted herbs, Pacific Botanicals emphasizes sustainable farming practices and environmental stewardship. Their selection includes many of the herbs used in Dr. Sebi's protocols, and they offer detailed information about the cultivation and harvesting processes. This transparency ensures that you are getting herbs that are not only effective but also ethically sourced.

In addition to these suppliers, another valuable resource is Frontier Co-op. Frontier Co-op is a cooperative business that focuses on natural and organic products. They offer a wide variety of herbs and spices, with a strong emphasis on quality and sustainability. Frontier Co-op's cooperative model also means that they are committed to fair trade practices and supporting the communities where their herbs are sourced. This ethical approach aligns with the holistic principles of Dr. Sebi's teachings.

While these suppliers are reputable, it's also beneficial to explore smaller, specialized herb shops and local growers. Farmers' markets often feature vendors who grow herbs organically and can provide valuable insights into their cultivation practices. Establishing a relationship with a local grower can offer the advantage of fresh, seasonal herbs that are often more potent and effective.

As you begin sourcing herbs, it's important to consider the forms in which they are available. Dried herbs are the most common and versatile, suitable for making teas, infusions, and capsules. Powders offer convenience and can be easily incorporated into smoothies and other foods. Liquid extracts and tinctures provide concentrated doses and are often preferred for their ease of use and rapid absorption. Understanding the different forms and their uses can help you make the best choices for your specific needs.

When purchasing herbs, always pay attention to the packaging and storage recommendations. Herbs should be stored in airtight containers away from light and moisture to preserve their potency. Suppliers who prioritize quality will often provide guidance on the best storage practices to ensure that their products remain effective.

In your search for reliable herb suppliers, it's also beneficial to leverage community resources. Online forums, social media groups, and natural health communities can offer recommendations and reviews from individuals who have firsthand experience with various suppliers. These personal testimonials can provide valuable insights and help you make informed decisions.

Ultimately, the key to successful sourcing of herbs lies in diligence and a commitment to quality. By choosing reputable suppliers and being mindful of storage and preparation methods, you can ensure that the herbs you use in your journey with Dr. Sebi's protocols are both effective and safe. These high-quality herbs will support your health goals and enhance your overall well-being, allowing you to fully experience the benefits of natural healing.

Recommended Further Reading and Studies

For anyone delving into Dr. Sebi's holistic approach to health, expanding your knowledge through further reading and studies can provide invaluable insights. This journey is not just about following a diet or using herbs; it's about understanding the science, history, and philosophy that underpin these practices. Fortunately, a wealth of resources is available to deepen your understanding and broaden your perspective.

One foundational book that complements Dr. Sebi's teachings is "The China Study" by T. Colin Campbell and Thomas M. Campbell II. This comprehensive study explores the relationship between diet and chronic disease, presenting compelling evidence that a plant-based diet can lead to better health outcomes. The authors detail extensive research conducted over several decades, highlighting the benefits of consuming whole, plant-based foods and the risks associated with animal-based products. This work provides a scientific backdrop that supports many of the principles advocated by Dr. Sebi, making it a valuable resource for those seeking to understand the broader implications of their dietary choices.

Another significant work is "How Not to Die" by Dr. Michael Greger. This book examines the leading causes of premature death and how diet and lifestyle changes can prevent them. Dr. Greger, a well-respected physician and advocate for plant-based nutrition, presents a detailed analysis of how certain foods can fight disease and promote longevity. His evidence-based approach aligns with the holistic principles of Dr. Sebi's diet, offering practical advice and scientific explanations that can enhance your journey towards better health. For those interested in the herbal aspect of Dr. Sebi's protocols, "The Earthwise Herbal: A Complete Guide to Old World Medicinal Plants" by Matthew Wood is an excellent resource. Wood, a renowned herbalist, provides detailed descriptions of various medicinal plants, their uses, and their healing properties. This guide is particularly useful for understanding the traditional uses of herbs and how they can be incorporated into modern health practices. Wood's holistic approach to herbal medicine resonates with Dr. Sebi's emphasis on natural remedies, making this book a valuable addition to your library. "The Alkaline Cure" by Dr. Stephan Domenig is another recommended read. This book explores the principles of the alkaline diet, offering practical guidance on how to implement it in your daily life. Dr. Domenig provides recipes, meal plans, and tips for maintaining an alkaline balance, all of which can help you navigate the dietary aspects of Dr. Sebi's protocols. His medical background and expertise lend credibility to the discussion, making it easier to understand the health benefits of an alkaline lifestyle.

For a deeper understanding of the body's detoxification processes, "Clean" by Dr. Alejandro Junger is a must-read. Dr. Junger, a cardiologist, and detoxification expert, explains how modern living can lead to toxin buildup in the body and how a structured detox program can restore health. His approach to cleansing aligns with Dr. Sebi's emphasis on detoxification as a key component of healing. This book provides practical detox strategies and emphasizes the importance of a clean, plant-based diet in maintaining overall health.

"The Blue Zones Solution" by Dan Buettner offers another valuable perspective. Buettner's research into the world's longest-lived communities reveals common dietary and lifestyle practices that contribute to longevity. Many of these practices, such as consuming a predominantly plant-based diet, align with Dr. Sebi's teachings. By exploring the habits of these "Blue Zones," you can gain insights into the practical applications of a healthy lifestyle and how it can promote longevity and vitality.For a more technical exploration of plant-based nutrition, "Becoming Vegan: The Complete Reference to Plant-Based Nutrition" by Brenda Davis and Vesanto Melina is highly recommended. This comprehensive guide covers all aspects of vegan nutrition, from macronutrients to micronutrients, and provides evidence-based recommendations for achieving optimal health on a plant-based diet. The authors, both registered dietitians, offer a detailed and scientifically grounded discussion that can enhance your understanding of the nutritional aspects of Dr. Sebi's diet.

For those interested in the historical and cultural context of herbal medicine, "The Lost Language of Plants" by Stephen Harrod Buhner is a fascinating read. Buhner explores the deep connection between humans and plants, emphasizing the importance of plant intelligence and communication. This book provides a broader perspective on the role of plants in human health and the environment, enriching your understanding of the herbal components of Dr. Sebi's protocols. To further explore the scientific research supporting plant-based diets and herbal medicine, academic journals such as "The Journal of Alternative and Complementary Medicine" and "Phytotherapy Research" offer peer-reviewed studies and articles. These journals provide the latest research findings and clinical studies on the efficacy of natural remedies, plant-based diets, and holistic health practices. Subscribing to these journals or accessing them through academic institutions can keep you updated on the latest developments in the field. In addition to books and academic journals, online resources such as the Plant-Based Nutrition Certificate offered by the T. Colin Campbell Center for Nutrition Studies can provide structured learning opportunities. This online course covers the science behind plant-based nutrition, offering lectures and resources from leading experts in the field. Completing this certificate program can deepen your knowledge and provide practical skills for implementing plant-based dietary practices.

Documentaries are another excellent way to gain insights into the benefits of plant-based diets and natural healing. Films such as "Forks Over Knives," "What the Health," and "The Game Changers" present compelling evidence and real-life stories of individuals who have transformed their health through dietary changes. These documentaries can inspire and educate, providing visual and emotional context to the principles discussed in Dr. Sebi's teachings. Lastly, engaging with online communities and forums dedicated to Dr. Sebi's diet and holistic health can offer support and additional resources. Websites like NutritionFacts.org, managed by Dr. Michael Greger, provide a wealth of information, including videos, articles, and research summaries on the benefits of plant-based nutrition. These platforms allow you to connect with like-minded individuals, share experiences, and access a broad range of information that can support your health journey.

By exploring these recommended readings and studies, you can deepen your understanding of Dr. Sebi's holistic health principles and the broader context of plant-based nutrition and herbal medicine. These resources offer valuable knowledge that can enhance your health journey and empower you to make informed decisions about your well-being.

Key Terms and Definitions

Embarking on a journey with Dr. Sebi's alkaline diet and herbal protocols can feel overwhelming at first, especially with the specialized terminology that accompanies this holistic approach. Understanding key terms and definitions is essential for fully grasping the principles and practices of Dr. Sebi's teachings. This guide aims to demystify the core vocabulary, providing clarity and enhancing your comprehension of the concepts central to this lifestyle.

At the heart of Dr. Sebi's philosophy is the concept of "alkalinity." The term "alkaline" refers to the pH level of substances, indicating their acidity or alkalinity on a scale from 0 to 14, with 7 being neutral. Substances with a pH above 7 are considered alkaline, while those below 7 are acidic. Dr. Sebi emphasized the importance of maintaining an alkaline state in the body to promote health and prevent disease. By consuming alkaline-forming foods and avoiding acidic ones, the body's pH balance can be optimized, reducing inflammation and fostering an environment less conducive to disease.

"pH balance" is another fundamental term, referring to the body's ability to maintain a stable pH level. The blood's pH is tightly regulated around 7.4, slightly alkaline. This balance is crucial for proper physiological function. The alkaline diet supports this balance by promoting foods that contribute to an alkaline internal environment, thereby aiding in various bodily processes, including detoxification and nutrient absorption.

The term "mucus" is frequently encountered in Dr. Sebi's teachings. He believed that excess mucus in the body is a root cause of many diseases. Mucus is a viscous secretion produced by mucous membranes, serving as a protective layer in various parts of the body. However, when mucus production is excessive, it can lead to congestion and inflammation. Dr. Sebi's diet aims to reduce mucus-producing foods, thereby alleviating conditions associated with excess mucus, such as respiratory and digestive issues.

"Detoxification," or "detox," is a process by which the body eliminates toxins. Dr. Sebi's protocols often include detoxification practices to cleanse the body of impurities that accumulate from environmental pollutants, processed foods, and other sources. Detoxification can involve fasting, consuming herbal teas, and following a strict alkaline diet. These practices support the liver, kidneys, and other detoxifying organs, enhancing the body's natural ability to purge harmful substances.

"Electric foods" is a term unique to Dr. Sebi's lexicon, referring to foods that are natural, unprocessed, and promote an alkaline state in the body. These foods are believed to carry a high level of bioelectricity, which is essential for cell function and overall vitality. Examples of electric foods include raw fruits, vegetables, nuts, and seeds that are free from genetic modification and industrial processing. Understanding "genetically modified organisms" (GMOs) is also crucial in the context of Dr. Sebi's diet. GMOs are organisms whose genetic material has been altered through genetic engineering. Dr. Sebi advocated for the consumption of non-GMO foods, arguing that natural, unaltered foods are more compatible with the human body's natural processes. Avoiding GMOs is a key aspect of adhering to the principles of natural, holistic health.

The term "wildcrafted" describes plants that are harvested from their natural, wild habitat rather than being cultivated on farms. Wildcrafted herbs are believed to be more potent and nutritious because they grow in their native environment, absorbing the natural minerals and nutrients from the soil. Dr. Sebi favored wildcrafted herbs for their purity and therapeutic efficacy, making them a cornerstone of his herbal protocols.

"Herbal infusions" are preparations made by steeping herbs in hot water to extract their beneficial compounds. This method is commonly used in Dr. Sebi's protocols to make teas that deliver the medicinal properties of various herbs. Infusions are a gentle way to consume herbs, allowing the body to absorb their nutrients and healing properties efficiently.

Another term often encountered is "herbal decoction." Unlike infusions, decoctions involve boiling herbs in water for an extended period, which is particularly effective for extracting the active ingredients from tougher plant materials such as roots and bark. Decoctions are a more concentrated form of herbal preparation, providing a potent means of delivering the therapeutic benefits of herbs.

"Fasting" is a practice central to many detoxification programs, including those recommended by Dr. Sebi. Fasting involves abstaining from all or certain types of food for a period, allowing the body to rest and heal. Types of fasting include water fasting, juice fasting, and fruit fasting, each with specific guidelines and benefits. Fasting can enhance the body's natural detox processes, improve digestion, and reset the metabolic system.

"Intracellular cleansing" is a term that highlights the importance of detoxifying at the cellular level. Dr. Sebi believed that true healing occurs within the cells, where toxins and waste products can accumulate and impede function. Intracellular cleansing involves practices that support the elimination of these toxins, such as consuming alkaline foods and herbs that facilitate cellular detoxification and regeneration.

"Mineral balance" is another critical concept, referring to the equilibrium of essential minerals in the body. Dr. Sebi emphasized the importance of consuming foods rich in natural minerals to maintain this balance, as minerals play vital roles in various physiological functions, including bone health, muscle function, and enzymatic reactions. Ensuring an adequate intake of minerals like calcium, magnesium, and potassium through diet and herbal supplements is a key aspect of maintaining overall health.

Lastly, the term "holistic health" encapsulates the philosophy underlying Dr. Sebi's teachings. Holistic health is an approach that considers the whole person—body, mind, and spirit—in the pursuit of wellness. It involves recognizing the interconnectedness of various aspects of health and addressing underlying causes of disease rather than just treating symptoms. Dr. Sebi's protocols are rooted in this holistic perspective, aiming to restore balance and harmony within the body through natural means.

Understanding these key terms and definitions is essential for anyone looking to adopt Dr. Sebi's alkaline diet and herbal practices. These concepts form the foundation of a holistic approach to health that emphasizes natural, unprocessed foods and the body's innate ability to heal. By familiarizing yourself with this vocabulary, you can navigate the principles and practices of Dr. Sebi's teachings with greater confidence and clarity, fully embracing the potential of natural healing.

Conclusion

As we reach the end of this exploration into the life, principles, and practices of Dr. Sebi, it's essential to reflect on the transformative potential that lies within the realm of natural health. The journey through Dr. Sebi's teachings is not just about adopting a new diet or trying out a few herbs; it's about embracing a holistic approach to wellness that fundamentally changes how we understand and interact with our bodies.

Dr. Sebi's philosophy emphasizes a return to nature, a reconnection with the earth's bounty that has sustained human life for millennia. In today's fast-paced, technologically driven world, this return is not merely a nostalgic longing for a simpler time but a vital step toward reclaiming our health. The rampant rise of chronic diseases, many of which are tied to lifestyle and dietary choices, signals a profound disconnection from natural ways of living. Dr. Sebi's approach serves as a reminder that the answers to many of our health challenges lie not in synthetic drugs or invasive procedures, but in the natural foods and herbs that have been available to us all along.

Embracing an alkaline diet as Dr. Sebi advocates involves more than just changing what's on our plates. It's a comprehensive shift in perspective, recognizing that food is not just fuel but medicine. This paradigm shift invites us to see each meal as an opportunity to nourish our bodies, to provide the essential nutrients that support our physiological functions, and to prevent and heal disease. By focusing on alkaline-forming foods, we can create an internal environment that promotes health, reduces inflammation, and fosters a state of balance and vitality.

Dr. Sebi's emphasis on the elimination of mucus as a key to health may initially seem simplistic, but it underscores a fundamental aspect of his teachings: the importance of addressing the root causes of disease rather than merely treating symptoms. This approach challenges the conventional medical paradigm that often prioritizes symptom management over true healing. By targeting the underlying factors that contribute to illness, such as dietary imbalances and toxin accumulation, Dr. Sebi's protocols aim to restore the body's natural equilibrium and enhance its ability to heal itself.

The role of herbs in Dr. Sebi's regimen cannot be overstated. These natural remedies, many of which have been used for centuries, offer potent healing properties that can complement and enhance the effects of an alkaline diet. Herbs such as burdock root, sarsaparilla, and bladderwrack provide specific benefits, from detoxification to immune support. Integrating these herbs into our daily routines not only addresses specific health concerns but also supports overall well-being by providing essential minerals and promoting detoxification.

As we've seen through the numerous success stories, the impact of Dr. Sebi's protocols can be profound and far-reaching. Individuals who have adopted his diet and herbal recommendations often report dramatic improvements in their health, from increased energy and mental clarity to the resolution of chronic conditions. These personal transformations highlight the power of natural healing and inspire others to explore these methods for themselves. The stories of healing and recovery serve as a testament to the efficacy of Dr. Sebi's approach and the resilience of the human body when given the proper support.

One of the most compelling aspects of Dr. Sebi's philosophy is its emphasis on self-empowerment. By educating ourselves about the foods and herbs that promote health, we take control of our well-being. This empowerment extends beyond individual health, fostering a broader movement toward community wellness and environmental stewardship. When we choose to consume natural, sustainably sourced foods and herbs, we support practices that are beneficial not only for our health but also for the planet. This holistic perspective aligns personal well-being with the health of our communities and the environment, creating a synergy that enhances life on multiple levels.

The journey of adopting Dr. Sebi's principles is not without challenges. It requires a commitment to change, a willingness to learn, and the courage to step away from conventional wisdom. The initial transition can be daunting, as it involves reevaluating long-held dietary habits and navigating the complexities of a new nutritional framework. However, the rewards of this journey are well worth the effort. As we align our diets with the principles of alkalinity and natural healing, we unlock the potential for vibrant health and longevity.

In embracing Dr. Sebi's teachings, we also reconnect with a broader tradition of holistic health practices that span cultures and centuries. Many of the principles he espoused are echoed in other traditional healing systems, from Ayurveda to Traditional Chinese Medicine. This cross-cultural resonance underscores the universality of natural healing principles and the timeless wisdom embedded in these practices. By integrating Dr. Sebi's approach with other holistic traditions, we can create a rich tapestry of health practices that draw on the best of multiple worlds.

Reflecting on the journey through this book, it becomes clear that Dr. Sebi's legacy is one of hope and possibility. His teachings offer a pathway to health that is accessible, natural, and profoundly transformative. Whether you are seeking to address specific health issues or simply looking to enhance your overall well-being, the principles of the alkaline diet and natural healing provide a robust framework for achieving your goals.

As you move forward, remember that the path to health is a continuous journey, not a destination. It involves ongoing learning, adaptation, and commitment. Embrace the process with curiosity and openness, and allow yourself to experiment and discover what works best for you. The principles outlined in Dr. Sebi's teachings are tools to guide you, but the ultimate power lies within you. By taking responsibility for your health and making informed choices, you can create a life of vitality, balance, and wellness.

In conclusion, Dr. Sebi's approach offers a compelling alternative to the conventional health paradigm. It invites us to return to nature, to harness the power of natural foods and herbs, and to embrace a holistic view of health that honors the interconnectedness of body, mind, and spirit. Through the adoption of an alkaline diet and the integration of healing herbs, we can transform our health and our lives. This journey requires dedication and perseverance, but the rewards are immeasurable. As we align ourselves with the principles of natural healing, we open the door to a future of optimal health and well-being.

Appendices

Appendix A: Nutritional Tables

Nutritional Values of Alkaline Foods

Understanding the nutritional values of alkaline foods is essential for anyone following Dr. Sebi's dietary principles. This knowledge not only helps you make informed choices about what you eat but also ensures that you are getting the necessary nutrients to maintain optimal health. Alkaline foods are primarily plant-based and include a variety of fruits, vegetables, nuts, seeds, and herbs. Each of these foods brings unique nutritional benefits that support the body's natural processes and promote overall well-being.

Let's begin with leafy greens, a cornerstone of the alkaline diet. Kale, for example, is not only alkaline-forming but also packed with vitamins A, C, and K. It's an excellent source of calcium, which is vital for bone health, and it provides a significant amount of fiber, which aids in digestion. Spinach is another leafy green that deserves attention. It is rich in iron, essential for oxygen transport in the blood, and contains magnesium, which supports muscle and nerve function.

Fruits, while naturally sweet, can also be highly alkaline-forming. Berries, such as strawberries, blueberries, and raspberries, are excellent examples. They are high in antioxidants, which protect the body from oxidative stress and inflammation. These fruits are also rich in vitamins C and E, contributing to skin health and immune function. Another fruit to consider is watermelon. Not only is it hydrating due to its high water content, but it also provides vitamins A and C and is known for its diuretic properties, helping the body flush out toxins.

Root vegetables like beets and sweet potatoes are also valuable additions to an alkaline diet. Beets are rich in folate, manganese, and potassium, and they have been shown to support liver function and improve blood circulation. Sweet potatoes, on the other hand, are an excellent source of beta-carotene, which the body converts to vitamin A, essential for vision and immune health. They also contain fiber, which promotes a healthy digestive system.

Nuts and seeds are another category of alkaline foods that provide a wealth of nutrients. Almonds, for instance, are rich in healthy fats, protein, and magnesium. They help balance blood sugar levels and support cardiovascular health. Chia seeds are another powerhouse, offering omega-3 fatty acids, fiber, and antioxidants. These seeds can aid in weight management by promoting a feeling of fullness and supporting digestive health.

Among herbs, those recommended by Dr. Sebi are particularly noted for their health benefits. Burdock root, for example, is known for its detoxifying properties. It is high in antioxidants and has been used traditionally to purify the blood and support liver health. Sarsaparilla is another herb with a strong nutritional profile. It contains saponins, which have anti-inflammatory and immune-boosting properties, and it is also rich in iron, aiding in the treatment of anemia and boosting energy levels.

Examining the nutritional profiles of alkaline foods reveals their potential to support various bodily functions. For instance, the high fiber content in many of these foods aids in digestion by promoting regular bowel movements and supporting gut health. Fiber is crucial for maintaining a healthy weight, as it helps you feel full longer, reducing overall calorie intake. Moreover, fiber-rich foods help control blood sugar levels by slowing the absorption of sugar into the bloodstream, which can be beneficial for individuals managing diabetes.

Vitamins and minerals found in alkaline foods play critical roles in maintaining health. Vitamin A, abundant in sweet potatoes and leafy greens, is vital for maintaining healthy vision, skin, and immune function. Vitamin C, found in berries and citrus fruits, is essential for collagen production, wound healing, and the absorption of iron from plant-based foods. Vitamin K, present in leafy greens like kale and spinach, is necessary for blood clotting and bone health.

Magnesium, another essential mineral, is found in abundance in nuts, seeds, and leafy greens. It supports muscle and nerve function, regulates blood pressure, and contributes to bone health. Potassium, which is plentiful in fruits like bananas and vegetables like beets, helps regulate fluid balance, muscle contractions, and nerve signals. Adequate potassium intake is also linked to a reduced risk of stroke and improved cardiovascular health.

Iron, a crucial component of hemoglobin, the protein in red blood cells that carries oxygen throughout the body, is found in various alkaline foods such as spinach, quinoa, and sarsaparilla. Ensuring sufficient iron intake is vital for preventing anemia and maintaining energy levels. Plant-based sources of iron are particularly important for those following a vegetarian or vegan diet.

The antioxidants found in many alkaline foods protect the body from damage caused by free radicals, unstable molecules that can lead to chronic diseases and aging. Antioxidants such as vitamin C, vitamin E, and beta-carotene neutralize free radicals, reducing oxidative stress and lowering the risk of chronic diseases such as heart disease, cancer, and neurodegenerative disorders. Berries, nuts, seeds, and leafy greens are particularly rich in these protective compounds.

Additionally, the diuretic properties of certain alkaline foods, such as watermelon and cucumber, help the body eliminate excess fluids and toxins, supporting kidney function and reducing blood pressure. These foods also promote hydration, which is crucial for maintaining all bodily functions, from digestion to temperature regulation.

Incorporating a variety of alkaline foods into your diet ensures that you receive a broad spectrum of nutrients necessary for optimal health. This diversity not only supports physical well-being but also enhances mental health by providing essential nutrients that support brain function and mood regulation. Omega-3 fatty acids from chia seeds and walnuts, for example, are known to support cognitive function and reduce the risk of depression.

Ultimately, understanding the nutritional values of alkaline foods enables you to make informed dietary choices that align with Dr. Sebi's principles. By focusing on nutrient-dense, plant-based foods, you can support your body's natural healing processes, maintain a balanced pH, and achieve a state of holistic health. The comprehensive benefits of these foods underscore the profound impact that diet has on overall well-being, highlighting the importance of integrating these principles into daily life. Through mindful eating and a commitment to natural foods, you can cultivate a vibrant, healthy life grounded in the wisdom of nature.

Comparison Table of Alkaline and Acidic Foods

To provide a clear visual representation of the nutritional differences between alkaline and acidic foods, below is a detailed comparison table. This table highlights key nutritional components and benefits of select foods from each category, illustrating the advantages of incorporating alkaline foods into your diet.

Food Category	Alkaline Foods	Nutritional Benefits	Acidic Foods	Nutritional Concerns
Leafy Greens	Kale	High in vitamins A, C, and K; rich in calcium, iron, and antioxidants	Tomatoes	High in vitamins A and C, but acidic, can cause heartburn in sensitive individuals
	Spinach	Excellent source of iron, magnesium, and fiber	Potatoes	Provides potassium and vitamin C, but higher in carbohydrates and can raise blood sugar levels
Fruits	Berries (Blueberries, Strawberries, Raspberries)	Rich in antioxidants, vitamins C and K, and fiber	Oranges	High in vitamin C, but acidic, can contribute to acid reflux
	Melons (Watermelon, Cantaloupe)	Hydrating, high in vitamins A and C, low in calories	Grapes	Contains antioxidants and vitamins, but higher acidity and sugar content
Nuts and Seeds	Almonds	High in healthy fats, protein, magnesium, and vitamin E	Peanuts	Contains protein and healthy fats, but more acidic and can cause allergies
	Chia Seeds	Rich in omega-3 fatty acids, fiber, and antioxidants	Sunflower Seeds	High in healthy fats and vitamin E, but can be acid-forming when consumed in large amounts

Food Category	Alkaline Foods	Nutritional Benefits	Acidic Foods	Nutritional Concerns
Root Vegetables	Beets	High in folate, manganese, and nitrates, supports liver function and blood circulation	White Potatoes	Good source of potassium and vitamin C, but higher glycemic index
	Sweet Potatoes	Rich in beta-carotene, vitamin C, and fiber	Carrots	High in beta-carotene and fiber, but can be more acid-forming
Grains	Quinoa	Complete protein, rich in fiber, iron, magnesium, and manganese	Wheat	Provides protein and fiber, but more acid-forming and can cause gluten sensitivity
	Amaranth	High in protein, fiber, iron, and calcium	White Rice	Provides energy, but higher glycemic index and lacks essential nutrients
Herbs	Burdock Root	Detoxifying properties, supports liver health, rich in antioxidants	Black Pepper	Contains antioxidants, but can be irritating to the gastrointestinal tract in large amounts
	Sarsaparilla	Anti-inflammatory, immune-boosting, rich in iron	Mustard Seeds	Contains antioxidants and vitamins, but more acid-forming
Dairy Alternatives	Almond Milk	Low in calories, rich in vitamins D and E,	Cow's Milk	High in calcium and protein, but more acid-forming and can

Food Category	Alkaline Foods	Nutritional Benefits	Acidic Foods	Nutritional Concerns
		supports bone and skin health		cause lactose intolerance
	Coconut Milk	Provides healthy fats and vitamins, supports hydration and digestion	Cheese	High in protein and calcium, but highly acidic and can contribute to inflammation
Beverages	Herbal Teas (Chamomile, Peppermint)	Soothing, antioxidant-rich, supports hydration without adding acidity	Coffee	Contains antioxidants, but highly acidic and can lead to dehydration and acid reflux
	Alkaline Water	Maintains body's pH balance, supports hydration and detoxification	Sodas	High in sugar and acidity, can lead to dehydration and long-term health issues

Summary

This comparison table clearly illustrates the nutritional superiority of alkaline foods over their acidic counterparts. Alkaline foods not only provide essential vitamins, minerals, and antioxidants but also support the body's natural pH balance, reducing inflammation and promoting overall health. By incorporating a variety of these nutrient-dense, alkaline-forming foods into your diet, you can enhance your well-being and prevent many of the health issues associated with a more acidic diet.

Making informed dietary choices by understanding the nutritional benefits and drawbacks of various foods is a crucial step in adopting a holistic approach to health. This table serves as a useful reference for anyone looking to optimize their diet in alignment with Dr. Sebi's principles, fostering a healthier, more balanced lifestyle.

Appendix B: Scientific References

Studies and research supporting Dr. Sebi's theories

Studies and Research Supporting Dr. Sebi's Theories

Dr. Sebi's holistic approach to health and wellness, rooted in the principles of an alkaline diet and natural healing, has garnered considerable attention. While his methods have been both celebrated and scrutinized, various scientific studies and research support several aspects of his theories. These studies provide a broader understanding of the benefits of an alkaline diet, the use of specific herbs, and the holistic health approach that Dr. Sebi advocated.

One core element of Dr. Sebi's approach is the emphasis on an alkaline diet. The theory is that maintaining an alkaline internal environment can promote better health and prevent disease. Research has shown that diet-induced acidosis, resulting from consuming a diet high in acid-forming foods, can contribute to several health issues. For instance, a study published in the "Journal of Environmental and Public Health" found that a diet rich in acid-forming foods could lead to decreased bone density, increased risk of hypertension, and the development of kidney stones. Conversely, the consumption of alkaline-forming foods was associated with improved bone health, reduced muscle wasting, and better cardiovascular health.

A notable aspect of the alkaline diet is its emphasis on plant-based foods, which are naturally alkaline. Numerous studies have highlighted the benefits of a plant-based diet. For example, a study published in "Nutrients" explored the impact of plant-based diets on cardiovascular health. The findings indicated that such diets are associated with lower blood pressure, improved cholesterol levels, and a reduced risk of heart disease. These results align with Dr. Sebi's assertion that an alkaline, plant-based diet can enhance overall health and prevent chronic diseases.

The role of specific herbs in promoting health is another crucial component of Dr. Sebi's philosophy. Herbs like burdock root, sarsaparilla, and bladderwrack are frequently mentioned in his protocols for their purported healing properties. Scientific research supports the use of these herbs for various health benefits. Burdock root, for instance, has been studied for its antioxidant and anti-inflammatory properties. A study in the "International Journal of Rheumatic Diseases" found that burdock root significantly reduced inflammatory markers in patients with osteoarthritis, supporting its use as a natural anti-inflammatory agent.

Similarly, sarsaparilla has been recognized for its medicinal properties. A study published in the "Journal of Ethnopharmacology" examined the anti-inflammatory and immune-boosting effects of sarsaparilla. The research demonstrated that sarsaparilla contains compounds that inhibit inflammatory processes and enhance immune function, validating its use in traditional medicine for treating inflammation and immune-related disorders.

Bladderwrack, another herb recommended by Dr. Sebi, is rich in iodine and other essential minerals. Research has shown that bladderwrack can support thyroid health due to its high iodine content. A study in the "Journal of Medicinal Food" highlighted bladderwrack's potential to improve thyroid function and support metabolic health. The study's findings suggest that bladderwrack can be beneficial for individuals with thyroid imbalances, corroborating Dr. Sebi's recommendation of this herb for thyroid support.

Detoxification is a significant theme in Dr. Sebi's protocols. He emphasized the importance of cleansing the body to remove toxins and promote healing. Scientific literature supports the concept that detoxification can enhance health. For instance, a review in the "Journal of Human Nutrition and Dietetics" discussed the benefits of dietary detoxification, noting that detox diets can help eliminate toxins, improve liver function, and support overall well-being. The review highlighted the role of specific foods and herbs in facilitating detoxification processes, aligning with Dr. Sebi's approach to using natural methods for cleansing the body.

Moreover, the concept of reducing inflammation through diet and herbs is well-supported by scientific research. Chronic inflammation is linked to various diseases, including heart disease, diabetes, and cancer. Studies have shown that an anti-inflammatory diet, rich in fruits, vegetables, nuts, seeds, and herbs, can significantly reduce inflammation and lower the risk of these chronic conditions. For example, a study published in the "American Journal of Clinical Nutrition" found that a diet high in anti-inflammatory foods was associated with lower levels of inflammatory markers and a reduced risk of chronic diseases. These findings support Dr. Sebi's emphasis on using natural, anti-inflammatory foods and herbs to promote health and prevent disease.

The holistic approach to health, considering the interconnectedness of diet, herbs, and overall lifestyle, is another cornerstone of Dr. Sebi's philosophy. This approach is increasingly supported by integrative and holistic health research. For instance, a study in "Global Advances in Health and Medicine" explored the benefits of holistic health practices, including dietary interventions, herbal medicine, and lifestyle changes. The research indicated that holistic approaches could effectively address multiple aspects of health, including physical, mental, and emotional well-being. The study's findings highlight the efficacy of holistic health strategies in promoting comprehensive wellness, echoing Dr. Sebi's holistic approach.

Furthermore, the role of diet in influencing body pH and overall health is a topic of ongoing research. While the body tightly regulates blood pH, dietary choices can affect urinary pH and the body's acid-base balance. A study in the "British Journal of Nutrition" examined the impact of an alkaline diet on health and found that such a diet could reduce the risk of chronic diseases, improve mineral balance, and enhance overall health. These findings support the idea that an alkaline diet, as advocated by Dr. Sebi, can have significant health benefits.

In addition to these scientific studies, ongoing research continues to explore the mechanisms behind the health benefits of an alkaline diet and the use of specific herbs. Advances in nutritional science and herbal medicine are increasingly validating the principles underlying Dr. Sebi's theories. As more studies are conducted, the body of evidence supporting natural, holistic health approaches continues to grow, providing further support for the effectiveness of Dr. Sebi's protocols.

In conclusion, the scientific literature provides substantial support for many aspects of Dr. Sebi's theories. The benefits of an alkaline diet, the therapeutic properties of specific herbs, and the holistic approach to health are well-documented in scientific research. These studies underscore the potential of natural, plant-based diets and herbal remedies to promote health, prevent disease, and enhance overall well-being. By integrating these principles into daily life, individuals can harness the power of natural healing and achieve a state of holistic wellness.

QR CODE

Thank you for reading "The Ultimate Dr. Sebi Encyclopedia." To help you get started on your journey toward optimal health, we've included a QR code at the end of this book. Scan it to download a comprehensive 60-day meal plan tailored to Dr. Sebi's alkaline diet principles.

Your feedback is invaluable to us. Please consider leaving a review to share your experience and help others discover the benefits of Dr. Sebi's holistic approach. Your thoughts and insights are greatly appreciated!

Made in the USA
Columbia, SC
21 June 2024

37345902R00096